Motivational Interviewing Techniques for Nurses

A comprehensive guide for Engaging Patients in Health Behavior Change

Honor Victoria Frost and Clarissa Mary Fernandez

© 2025 Honor Victoria Frost and Clarissa Mary Fernandez

All rights reserved. No part of this publication may be reproduced, distributed, or transmitted in any form or by any means, including photocopying, recording, or other electronic or mechanical methods, without the prior written permission of the publisher, except in the case of brief quotations embodied in critical reviews and certain other noncommercial uses permitted by copyright law.

ISBN: 978-1-923370-48-7
Isohan Publishing

Disclaimer: Although the publisher and authors have made every effort to ensure that the information in this book was correct at press time, the publisher and authors do not assume and hereby disclaim any liability to any party for any loss, damage, or disruption caused by errors or omissions, or for the application or misuse of information contained in this book.

The information presented in this book, "Motivational Interviewing Techniques for Nurses: Engaging Patients in Health Behavior Change," is intended for educational and informational purposes only. The content is designed to support nurses and other healthcare professionals in developing communication skills related to Motivational Interviewing within a clinical context.

This book does not constitute medical advice, nor is it intended to replace or substitute for professional medical advice, diagnosis, or treatment. Always seek the advice of a qualified healthcare provider with any questions you may have regarding a medical condition or treatment plan. Never disregard professional medical advice or delay in seeking it because of something you have read in this book.

The principles and techniques described are based on the authors' interpretation and application of Motivational Interviewing within nursing practice. Healthcare is constantly evolving, and standards of care may change. Readers are encouraged to consult current professional guidelines, institutional policies, and relevant research to ensure their practice aligns with the latest evidence and standards. Individual patient situations vary greatly, and clinical judgment must always be applied when interacting with patients.

Any case studies, examples, or patient scenarios presented in this book are illustrative. While inspired by clinical experience, patient details have been significantly altered, anonymised, or are composites created for educational purposes to protect confidentiality and privacy. They do not represent any specific individual.

Table of Contents

Preface 5

The Nurse's Crucial Role in Change 8

Chapter 1: The MI Mindset-The Spirit and Principles in Nursing Practice 19

Chapter 2: Your MI Toolkit- Mastering the Core Skills (OARS) in Minutes 33

Chapter 3: Listening for Change-Recognizing and Responding to Change Talk 48

Chapter 4: Dancing with Discord-Navigating Ambivalence and Rolling with Resistance 62

Chapter 5: Sharing Information Effectively-The Elicit-Provide-Elicit (EPE) Method 75

Chapter 6: From Talk to Action-Collaborative Goal Setting and Planning 87

Chapter 7: CMI in Motion- Applying Techniques in Common Nursing Scenarios 99

Chapter 8: Adding MI into Your Workflow-Tips for Time-Constrained Encounters 112

Chapter 9: Sustaining Your Practice-Self-Reflection and Preventing Burnout 124

Chapter 10: Case Studies Applying MI Across Nursing Settings 138

Appendices 163

References 166

Preface

If you are a nurse working in almost any setting—from the fast pace of primary care or hospital wards to the community outreach of public health or the specialised focus of mental health or chronic disease management—you know this truth: a significant part of your work involves talking with people about change. Changing habits, changing perspectives, changing how they manage their health. You educate, you advise, you encourage, you support. And sometimes, despite your best efforts and clearest explanations, you watch patients struggle to translate good intentions into sustained action. That can be deeply frustrating, both for the patient and for you.

We—the authors—have spent years working within and alongside nursing, training healthcare professionals in communication approaches designed to make those conversations about change less frustrating and more productive. We've seen firsthand the dedication nurses bring to their roles, and also the very real pressures of time constraints, heavy workloads, and the emotional weight of caring for people facing difficult health challenges.

This book, **Motivational Interviewing Techniques for Nurses: Engaging Patients in Health Behaviour Change**, grew directly from those experiences. We saw a need for a resource that specifically addresses how nurses can effectively use the principles and core techniques of Motivational Interviewing (MI) within the unique context of their practice. MI, as you will discover, isn't about magic tricks or complicated psychological theories. It is fundamentally a **collaborative conversation style** designed to strengthen a person's own motivation and commitment to change. It's about shifting from a traditional dynamic—where the nurse might feel responsible for *fixing* the patient or *persuading* them to change—to one of partnership, where you skillfully guide the patient to explore their *own* reasons, their *own* ambivalence, and their *own* path forward.

Our goal here is explicitly **practical**. We know you don't have time for dense academic texts or lengthy theoretical arguments. You need tools you can understand quickly and apply effectively, perhaps even in those brief "fly-by" moments during a busy shift. Therefore, this book focuses on the **core elements** of MI: the underlying spirit (that collaborative, accepting, compassionate, evocative stance), the essential OARS communication skills (Open questions, Affirmations, Reflections, Summaries), and practical strategies for common situations like navigating resistance, sharing information (using Elicit-Provide-Elicit), and helping patients build actionable plans.

We've consciously chosen to emphasise application over abstract theory. You will find numerous **nursing-specific examples and case studies** throughout these pages, illustrating how MI can sound and feel in conversations about medication adherence, lifestyle adjustments, managing chronic conditions, dealing with low motivation, and other everyday scenarios. We've tried to demonstrate how MI can be woven into your existing workflow—not as an extra burden, but as a way to make the communication you already do more efficient and effective in the long run. Reducing arguments and increasing patient buy-in can, perhaps counterintuitively, save time and emotional energy.

This book is written for you—the dedicated nurse seeking ways to enhance your communication skills, improve patient engagement, support adherence more effectively, and ultimately, find even greater satisfaction in your essential work. It requires a shift in perspective, certainly, and practice to become comfortable with the skills. But it's a shift grounded in respect for the patient and aligned with the core values of compassionate nursing care.

We hope this guide serves as a clear, accessible, and useful resource on your journey toward incorporating Motivational Interviewing into your practice. We believe it offers a powerful way to help your patients harness their own potential for change, leading to better health outcomes and stronger therapeutic relationships.

Honor Victoria Frost and Clarissa Mary Fernandez

The Nurse's Crucial Role in Change

Why MI Matters (and Why It's Practical)

You stand at a unique intersection in healthcare. Every shift, every patient interaction, places you in a position not just to treat illness, but to influence health. You are the educator, the supporter, the listener, the constant presence during moments of vulnerability and decision-making. From the organized chaos of an emergency department to the quiet continuity of a primary care clinic, from the specialized focus of chronic disease management to the sensitive work in mental health or the outreach in community settings—your role is fundamental. You see patients navigate complex medication regimens, grapple with life-altering diagnoses, and contemplate changes to long-held habits. You are there.

And because you are there, you also witness the human side of health behavior change—or the lack thereof. You experience the rewards, certainly. There's immense satisfaction in seeing a patient successfully manage their diabetes through lifestyle adjustments you discussed, or watching someone finally quit smoking after months of conversation, or helping a new parent gain confidence in caring for their infant. These moments fuel the dedication that defines nursing. They are the bright spots, the affirmations of why you entered this demanding profession.

But let's be direct—it's not always rewarding. Alongside the successes are the daily challenges, the encounters that leave you feeling perplexed, concerned, maybe even a little exasperated. These aren't failures of care, but rather the complex realities of human behavior meeting the demands of health management.

The Weight of Unanswered Questions

Think about your recent shifts. Did you meticulously explain the importance of taking blood pressure medication, only to have the patient return with dangerously high readings, admitting they "forgot" or didn't think it was necessary? Did you spend time reviewing dietary guidelines with someone newly diagnosed with heart failure, providing clear handouts and answering questions, yet their food diary later revealed choices directly counter to your advice? Perhaps you worked with an individual struggling with addiction, offering resources and encouragement, but saw them return to familiar patterns.

These situations are common—painfully common. You might find yourself thinking, *"I laid it all out so clearly. They seemed to understand. Why aren't they doing what's good for them?"* Or perhaps, *"I've told Mr. Henderson about his smoking risks a dozen times. What more can I possibly say?"* This feeling, this subtle or sometimes not-so-subtle frustration, isn't a sign of poor nursing. It's a sign that the traditional approach of **giving information** and **expecting action** often falls short when it comes to behavior change.

People aren't empty vessels waiting to be filled with our expert advice. They come with their own beliefs, fears, priorities, past experiences, and levels of confidence. Simply telling someone *what* to do, even with the best intentions and the clearest explanations, often bumps up against their internal ambivalence—that state of feeling two ways about something. *"Yes, I know I should quit smoking,* **but** *it helps me relax." "I want to lose weight,* **but** *I don't have time to exercise." "Taking that medication every day is probably smart,* **but** *I hate the side effects and I feel fine right now."*

This "yes, but..." is the heart of ambivalence, and directly confronting it, telling people why their "but" is wrong, usually just makes them dig their heels in deeper. We call this the "righting reflex"—our natural inclination as helpers to fix problems and offer solutions. Unfortunately, when it comes to behavior change, jumping in to "fix it" often backfires. Consider this typical scenario:

Nurse Davis and Mr. Chen

Nurse Davis works in a busy primary care clinic. Mr. Chen, a 58-year-old man with Type 2 diabetes and hypertension, is in for a routine follow-up. His A1c is elevated again, despite Nurse Davis having reviewed his diet and medication adherence plan three months prior.

Nurse Davis: "Mr. Chen, your A1c is 9.2 percent today. That's quite a bit higher than we'd like. We talked last time about cutting back on sugary drinks and checking your blood sugar regularly. Have you been able to do that?"

Mr. Chen: (Looks down) "Well, I try, but it's hard. Work has been stressful, and sometimes I just grab a soda. And checking my sugar... I forget sometimes."

Nurse Davis: "Mr. Chen, forgetting isn't really an option with diabetes. High blood sugar can lead to serious problems—nerve damage, kidney failure, even blindness. You really need to prioritize checking your levels and avoiding those sodas. Maybe keep your meter by your toothbrush so you remember in the morning?"

Mr. Chen: "Yeah, I guess. But the mornings are so rushed." (He shifts uncomfortably). "And the sodas... it's just one thing I enjoy."

Nurse Davis: "Enjoying soda isn't worth losing your eyesight, is it? We need to get this A1c down. I'm going to give you these pamphlets again, and let's schedule another follow-up sooner, in one month, to see if you've made progress."

Mr. Chen leaves the clinic clutching the pamphlets, likely feeling lectured and perhaps a bit resentful. Nurse Davis feels frustrated, worried about Mr. Chen's health, and unsure what else she could have done. She provided clear information, highlighted the risks, and offered a solution (keep the meter by the toothbrush). Yet, the conversation felt unproductive, even strained. Mr. Chen didn't seem motivated; if anything, he seemed more resistant. This dynamic is exhausting for both parties and often leads nowhere productive.

A Different Way: Introducing Motivational Interviewing (MI)

What if Nurse Davis had approached that conversation differently? What if, instead of immediately focusing on the high A1c and telling Mr. Chen what he *needed* to do, she explored *his* perspective first? This is where Motivational Interviewing offers a path forward.

Motivational Interviewing isn't a technique to *make* people change. It's a **guiding communication style** designed to help people explore their *own* reasons for change and resolve that internal ambivalence we talked about. It's collaborative, person-centered, and respects patient autonomy—their right to make their own choices, even choices we might disagree with.

Think of it less like wrestling—where you try to pin down resistance—and more like dancing—where you move *with* the person, responding to their cues, guiding gently, and working together.

Now, hearing "interviewing" might conjure images of lengthy, structured sessions. Let's clear that up immediately. While MI originated in counseling settings, its principles and core skills are remarkably adaptable. This book is **not** about turning you into a therapist or adding another hour-long task to your already packed schedule. It's about integrating specific MI communication skills and its underlying "spirit" into the interactions you *already* have with patients. It's about making those brief moments—during an assessment, while giving medications, during discharge teaching—more impactful.

MI operates on a few key ideas:

1. **People possess their own arguments for change:** Our job isn't to *give* them reasons, but to help them *find* and *voice* their own. Mr. Chen likely already knows soda isn't great for his diabetes; the motivation has to connect with something *he* values (like maybe having energy to play with his grandkids, rather than just avoiding blindness).

2. **Ambivalence is normal:** Feeling stuck between wanting to change and wanting things to stay the same is part of the process. MI helps explore both sides without judgment.

3. **Direct persuasion is often ineffective:** Pushing against resistance usually strengthens it. Rolling *with* resistance, acknowledging the person's perspective, is more productive.

4. **The therapeutic relationship matters:** A trusting, collaborative partnership between nurse and patient is the foundation for change.

Using MI doesn't mean abandoning your clinical expertise or failing to provide necessary information. It means changing *how* you have those conversations. It means asking more open-ended questions, listening reflectively to understand the patient's world, affirming their strengths and efforts, and offering information in a way they can actually hear and use.

Tailored for Your World: MI in Nursing Practice

You work in a unique environment. Time is often short. Patient needs are diverse and complex. You juggle multiple tasks simultaneously. Any communication approach needs to be flexible, efficient, and applicable across various settings and acuity levels.

That's precisely the focus of this book. We will translate the core components of MI into practical strategies that fit the realities of nursing:

- **Primary Care:** Engaging patients in managing chronic conditions like hypertension, diabetes, asthma; discussing preventative screenings; addressing lifestyle factors like diet, exercise, smoking, or alcohol use during brief office visits.

- **Community Health:** Working with diverse populations on health promotion, connecting individuals with resources, building trust with marginalized groups, supporting long-term behavior change goals.

- **Mental Health:** Collaborating with patients on medication adherence, addressing substance use, supporting engagement in therapy, building motivation for self-care and recovery goals.

- **Chronic Disease Management:** Helping patients navigate complex self-management tasks, cope with the emotional burden of illness, set realistic goals, and troubleshoot barriers to adherence over time.

- **Acute Care/Hospitals:** Discussing discharge plans, medication adherence post-hospitalization, addressing substance use identified during admission, motivating patients to engage in rehabilitation or follow-up care.

MI provides a framework that respects the patient while making your efforts more effective. It can help you navigate those challenging conversations—the ones about sensitive topics, low motivation, or apparent non-adherence—with greater skill and less frustration. It can, paradoxically, sometimes even save time in the long run by reducing resistance and the need for repetitive "lectures" that don't stick. When patients feel heard and understood, they are more likely to engage honestly and consider change.

The Promise of This Guide: Practical Skills, Real Examples, Respect for Your Time

My goal as an MI specialist and nurse advocate is simple: to equip you with practical, usable MI skills that you can begin applying immediately. This book is designed as a **concise, hands-on guide**, not an academic treatise.

Here's what you can expect:

1. **Focus on Core Skills:** We will concentrate on the fundamental elements of MI—the underlying spirit and the key communication techniques (often remembered by the acronym OARS: Open questions, Affirmations, Reflections, Summaries) that give you the most impact.

2. **Nursing-Specific Examples:** Forget generic counseling scenarios. We will use examples drawn directly from primary care, community health, mental health, and chronic disease management settings—situations you encounter regularly. You'll see how MI looks and sounds in conversations about medication, diet, appointments, self-monitoring, and more. We will explore detailed case examples, breaking down the dialogue to show MI in action.

3. **Emphasis on Practicality:** Theory is kept to a minimum. The focus is on *how* to integrate these skills into your existing workflow, even during brief interactions. We'll address the "how-to" for time-constrained environments.

4. **Actionable Strategies:** You'll get clear guidance on recognizing patient cues (like "change talk" – when they voice their own reasons for changing), responding effectively to resistance without arguing, and sharing information collaboratively using methods like "Elicit-Provide-Elicit."

5. **Respect for Your Expertise and Time:** This book acknowledges your professional knowledge and the pressures you face. MI is presented as a tool to *enhance* your practice, not overhaul it or add impossible burdens.

Consider again Nurse Davis and Mr. Chen. Using an MI approach might sound different:

Nurse Davis: (Warmly) "Mr. Chen, thanks for coming in. We got your lab results back, and your A1c is 9.2 percent today. That's higher than we were aiming for. What are your thoughts about that number?" (Open Question)

Mr. Chen: (Looks down) "Yeah, it's not good. I guess I haven't been doing great with the diet... or checking my sugars like I should."

Nurse Davis: "So you're recognizing that things haven't gone exactly as planned regarding your diet and blood sugar checks." (Simple Reflection) "It sounds like managing it all has been pretty challenging lately." (Complex Reflection – guessing at feeling)

Mr. Chen: "It really has. Work has been so stressful, just crazy hours. By the time I get home, I'm exhausted. Grabbing a soda is easy, and checking my sugar feels like one more thing I failed at."

Nurse Davis: "It takes a lot of effort to manage diabetes, especially when life throws extra stress your way. And it sounds like you're feeling discouraged when you can't keep up with it perfectly." (Affirmation of effort/Reflection of feeling) "Tell me a bit more about what makes checking your sugar feel like a chore right now?" (Open Question)

This conversation is just beginning, but notice the difference. Nurse Davis is exploring Mr. Chen's perspective, acknowledging his struggles without judgment, and reflecting his feelings. There's no lecture, no immediate "fix." Instead, she's building rapport and creating space for Mr. Chen to explore his *own* situation and, potentially, his *own* reasons for wanting things to be different. This approach is far more likely to engage Mr. Chen and lead to a collaborative plan he feels invested in. It requires skill, yes, but not necessarily more *time* than the original, less productive conversation. It redirects the energy toward understanding and collaboration.

This book is your guide to learning and applying that skill. It's about adding a powerful communication tool to your already extensive nursing toolkit—one that can make a real difference in your patients' lives and in your own professional satisfaction.

Key Insights from This Section

- Nurses are ideally positioned to influence patient health behaviors due to their frequent and trusted interactions.
- A common nursing frustration stems from the gap between providing health advice and seeing patients implement changes.
- Traditional information-giving often fails because it doesn't address a patient's internal ambivalence or readiness for change.
- Motivational Interviewing (MI) is a collaborative communication style, not a way to force change, that helps patients find their *own* motivation.
- MI focuses on partnership, acceptance, compassion, and evoking the patient's own ideas (PACE spirit).

- This guide translates MI principles into practical, time-efficient skills specifically for diverse nursing settings.
- The goal is to enhance existing nurse-patient conversations, making them more effective and less frustrating, even in brief encounters.

Now that we've established the 'why'—the critical need for more effective conversations about behavior change in nursing—let's move to the 'how.' The next step is to understand the foundational mindset, the "Spirit" of MI, that underpins all the techniques we will explore. This spirit is what transforms communication from directing to guiding.

Chapter 1: The MI Mindset-The Spirit and Principles in Nursing Practice

We've acknowledged the gap—the space between our well-intentioned advice and our patients' actions. We see the frustration it breeds, both for them and for us. Motivational Interviewing (MI) offers a different approach, a way to bridge that gap not by pushing harder, but by connecting differently. But before we get into specific techniques—the asking, the listening, the summarizing—we need to grasp the foundation upon which they are built. MI is more than just a set of skills; it's a way of *being* with patients. This underlying philosophy, often called the **"Spirit of MI,"** is what makes the techniques effective. Without the spirit, the techniques can feel hollow, mechanical, even manipulative. With it, they become powerful tools for fostering genuine collaboration and change.

Think of it like building a house. The OARS skills (Open questions, Affirmations, Reflections, Summaries) we'll discuss in the next chapter are the tools—the hammer, the saw, the level. But the Spirit of MI is the architectural plan and the solid foundation. You can have the best tools in the world, but without a good plan and a solid base, the structure won't be sound. Similarly, using MI techniques without embodying the spirit won't lead to meaningful, patient-centered change.

Beyond Techniques: The Heart of MI - The "Spirit" (PACE)

The Spirit of MI can be captured by the acronym **PACE**, representing four interwoven elements: Partnership, Acceptance, Compassion, and Evocation. Let's look closely at each one, considering what it means in the context of your busy nursing practice.

Partnership: Collaborating with the patient, not directing them

This is perhaps the most fundamental shift from traditional healthcare communication. In MI, the nurse and patient are collaborators. You are not the expert handing down instructions from on high; you are a knowledgeable guide working *alongside* the patient on their journey. The patient is recognized as the expert on their own life, their values, their challenges, and their motivations.

- **What it looks like:**
    - Asking permission before offering advice ("Would you be interested in hearing about some strategies other patients have found helpful?").
    - Using language that implies collaboration ("How might *we* approach this?" "What are *your* thoughts on the next step?").
    - Actively seeking the patient's input and ideas.
    - Avoiding jargon that creates a power imbalance.
    - Structuring the interaction as a shared exploration, not an interrogation or a lecture.
- **What it avoids:**
    - The "expert trap"—assuming you know best and simply need to impart your wisdom.

- Directing, demanding, or coercing.
- Taking primary responsibility for the patient's choices or outcomes. You are responsible for providing good care and facilitating the conversation; the patient is responsible for their decisions.

Consider Nurse Miller and Mrs. Jones: Mrs. Jones has frequently missed appointments for her diabetes check-ups.

- *Traditional (Directive) Approach:* "Mrs. Jones, you've missed three appointments. It's really important you come to these check-ups to manage your diabetes properly. You need to make these a priority."
- *MI Partnership Approach:* "Mrs. Jones, I notice you've had difficulty making it to your last few appointments. It can be tough juggling everything. What's been getting in the way for you?" (This opens a conversation, seeking her expertise on her own barriers). "How might we figure out a plan for follow-up that works better with your schedule?" (Invites collaboration on solutions).

Partnership sets a tone of respect and recognizes that lasting change comes from within the patient, not from external pressure. It empowers patients by involving them directly in their own care planning.

Acceptance: Recognizing autonomy, affirming strengths, accurate empathy, absolute worth

Acceptance is multifaceted. It doesn't necessarily mean *approval* of a patient's behavior (like smoking or not taking medications), but it does mean fundamentally accepting the person as they are, where they are. It has four key aspects:

1. **Absolute Worth:** Every patient has inherent value and deserves respect, regardless of their health status, behaviors, or circumstances. Your care is unconditional.

2. **Accurate Empathy:** This is the skill of actively trying to understand the patient's world from *their* perspective, without judgment. It's seeing the situation through their eyes, feeling it from their side (as best you can), and reflecting that understanding back to them.

3. **Autonomy Support:** Patients have the right to choose their own path, even if that path involves choices you disagree with or that carry health risks. Your role is to inform and support, not control. Forcing change rarely works and often damages the relationship. Acknowledging their right to choose ("Ultimately, the decision about whether or when you quit smoking is yours") can paradoxically make them *more* open to considering change.

4. **Affirmation:** Actively noticing and acknowledging the patient's strengths, resources, past successes, and efforts—no matter how small. This builds confidence and counteracts the discouragement that often accompanies struggling with behavior change. ("It took courage to even bring this up today." "You've managed to cut back before, which shows you have the ability.")

- **What it looks like:**

- Listening without interrupting or judging.
- Reflecting the patient's feelings and perspectives accurately ("So, it sounds like you're feeling overwhelmed by all these medication changes").
- Explicitly stating their right to choose ("It's up to you what you decide to do about this").
- Pointing out positive steps or qualities ("You've been very consistent about tracking your blood pressure this week, even with everything else going on").

- **What it avoids:**
    - Judgmental language or tone.
    - Trying to force agreement or compliance.
    - Focusing solely on problems or deficits.
    - Ignoring or dismissing the patient's perspective.

Acceptance creates a safe space for patients to be honest about their struggles and ambivalence without fear of being shamed or scolded. It's in this safe space that genuine exploration of change becomes possible.

Compassion: Actively promoting the other's welfare

This aligns closely with the core values of nursing. Compassion in MI means actively prioritizing the patient's well-being and acting in their best interests—as *they* perceive them, not just as *we* define them. It's the genuine commitment to understanding and supporting the patient's needs. It's the "why" behind the partnership and acceptance.

- **What it looks like:**
    - Expressing genuine concern for the patient's struggles.
    - Making choices in the conversation that serve the patient's goals, not your own agenda (like just getting through the checklist).
    - Being patient and understanding, even when progress is slow.
    - Advocating for the patient's needs within the healthcare system when appropriate.
- **What it avoids:**
    - Self-interest (e.g., rushing the conversation to save time).
    - Detachment or indifference.
    - Exploiting the patient's vulnerability.

Compassion ensures that MI is used ethically and effectively, always centered on the patient's welfare. It's the heart that fuels the helping relationship.

Evocation: Drawing out the patient's own reasons and ideas for change

This is where MI diverges sharply from directive approaches. Instead of *installing* motivation or *giving* solutions, you evoke them—you draw them out from *within* the patient. The assumption is that the patient already possesses arguments for change, resources, and ideas; your job is to help them discover and voice these.

- **What it looks like:**
    - Asking open-ended questions about the patient's values, goals, and concerns ("What are the things that matter most to you in your life right now?" "What worries you about your current situation?" "What are the good things about making this change?").
    - Listening intently for "change talk"—any statement the patient makes that favors movement toward a specific change.
    - Reflecting and summarizing the patient's own motivations ("So, being able to play with your grandkids without getting breathless is really important to you, and you see quitting smoking as a way to achieve that").
    - Asking about past successes or existing strengths related to the change ("What have you tried before that worked, even for a little while?").
- **What it avoids:**
    - Telling the patient why *they* should change.
    - Offering unsolicited advice or solutions.
    - Focusing only on the clinician's reasons for wanting the change.

Evocation empowers patients by connecting change to their own values and aspirations. People are much more likely to act on their *own* reasons than on reasons imposed upon them. When Mr. Chen connects managing his diabetes not just to avoiding complications (the nurse's concern) but to having energy for his woodworking hobby (his value), the motivation becomes internal and far more powerful.

Embodying PACE—Partnership, Acceptance, Compassion, and Evocation—creates a conversational atmosphere where patients feel respected, understood, and empowered to consider change. It's the fundamental mindset shift required for MI to be effective.

Core Principles Guiding Your Conversations

Flowing from the Spirit of MI are four guiding principles that help shape your interactions. These aren't rigid steps, but rather overlapping concepts that inform *how* you apply MI skills.

1. Expressing Empathy (It's more than just being nice)

We touched on accurate empathy under Acceptance. This principle emphasizes that demonstrating understanding is key. It involves skilled reflective listening—hearing not just the words but the underlying meaning and feeling, and reflecting that back to the patient. It's saying, in essence, "I hear you, I understand your perspective, even if I don't fully agree with it."

- **Why it matters:** When patients feel genuinely understood, they are more likely to open up, explore issues more deeply, and feel less defensive. It builds rapport and trust, the bedrock of any therapeutic relationship.

- **Nursing Focus:** Taking a moment to reflect a patient's feeling ("It sounds incredibly frustrating to deal with that side effect") before jumping to solutions can transform the interaction. It validates their experience.

2. Developing Discrepancy (Helping patients see the gap between goals and behavior)

MI aims to help patients see the mismatch—the discrepancy—between their current behavior and their deeply held values or future goals. This isn't about pointing fingers or inducing guilt. It's about helping the patient become aware of how their actions (e.g., smoking, skipping medication) might be taking them *away* from something they truly want (e.g., better health, more energy, being there for family).

- **How it works:** You evoke the patient's values and goals, and then juxtapose them with their current behavior, often using reflections or summaries. "So on one hand, feeling healthy and independent is really important to you, and on the other hand, continuing to smoke sometimes gets in the way of that. What do you make of that?"

- **Key:** The patient, not the nurse, should be the one making the argument for change based on this perceived discrepancy. Your role is to facilitate their awareness.

- **Nursing Focus:** Linking adherence to medication not just to lab numbers, but to the patient's stated desire to attend their daughter's wedding feeling well. "You mentioned wanting to feel your best for the wedding in June. How does managing your blood pressure fit into that picture for you?"

3. Rolling with Resistance (Avoiding the "righting reflex" and arguments)

Resistance—or more accurately termed "discord" in the relationship—is a signal. It often indicates that the patient feels pushed, misunderstood, or that their autonomy is threatened. The natural (but unhelpful) reaction is the "righting reflex"—to argue, persuade, correct, or take the opposing side. MI teaches us to "roll with" this discord instead of fighting against it.

- **Strategies:**
    - **Simple Reflection:** Reflecting the patient's statement of resistance without judgment ("You don't think this medication is really necessary right now").
    - **Shifting Focus:** Moving the conversation away from the sticking point temporarily.
    - **Reframing:** Offering a different interpretation of the situation ("Maybe it's not about lack of willpower, but about finding a strategy that fits better into your busy life").
    - **Emphasizing Personal Choice:** Explicitly affirming their autonomy ("Ultimately, it's your decision what you do").
- **Why it matters:** Arguing usually just entrenches the patient in their position. Rolling with resistance avoids confrontation, respects autonomy, and keeps the door open for further conversation.

- **Nursing Focus:** When a patient says, "These dietary changes are impossible," instead of saying "No, they're not, you just need to try harder," try reflecting: "It feels completely overwhelming to think about changing how you eat right now." This validates their feeling and makes them less likely to shut down.

4. Supporting Self-Efficacy (Building patient confidence in their ability to change)

Change is hard. Patients often lack confidence in their ability to succeed, especially if they've tried and failed before. Supporting self-efficacy means believing in the patient's capacity to change and actively helping them build their own confidence.

- **How it's done:**
    - **Affirming strengths and past successes:** ("You managed to walk three times last week, even when the weather wasn't great. That shows real determination.")
    - **Highlighting small steps and progress.**
    - **Expressing confidence in their ability:** ("I believe you have what it takes to figure this out.")
    - **Reframing past "failures" as learning experiences.**
    - **Helping them break down large goals into manageable steps.**
- **Why it matters:** Belief in one's ability to change (self-efficacy) is a strong predictor of actual change. If

patients don't believe they *can* do it, they likely won't even try.

- **Nursing Focus:** When teaching a complex self-care task (like using an inhaler or checking blood sugar), focus not just on the steps but on building the patient's confidence. "You picked that up really quickly. What helped you learn it so well?" Affirm their capability.

Nursing Focus: How the MI Spirit Transforms Brief Patient Interactions

Adopting the MI spirit and keeping these principles in mind doesn't require lengthy sessions. It transforms the *quality* of even brief encounters. When you approach a patient with **Partnership**, you invite collaboration from the start. When you practice **Acceptance** and **Compassion**, you create safety and trust. When you focus on **Evocation**, you tap into the patient's own wellspring of motivation.

Imagine a quick medication check-in.

- *Without MI Spirit:* "Are you taking your Lisinopril every day like you're supposed to?" (Closed question, implies judgment if the answer is no).
- *With MI Spirit:* "How has it been going with taking the Lisinopril each day?" (Open question - Partnership). The patient says, "Okay, but I miss it sometimes." You respond, "It can be tough to get into a new routine." (Accurate Empathy - Acceptance). "What helps you remember on the days you do take it?" (Evocation, focusing on strengths).

Or a brief encounter about smoking:

- *Without MI Spirit:* "You know you really need to quit smoking, right? It's terrible for your COPD." (Directive, potential for resistance).

- *With MI Spirit:* "We've talked about smoking before. What are your thoughts about it these days?" (Open question, Partnership, respects Autonomy). Patient expresses ambivalence. You reflect both sides: "So part of you knows it affects your breathing, but another part really relies on it for stress." (Accurate Empathy, develops Discrepancy gently). "What might be a small step you'd even *consider* related to smoking right now?" (Evocation, supports Self-Efficacy for small steps).

These aren't extended counseling sessions. They are subtle shifts in language and approach, guided by PACE and the core principles, that make routine interactions more collaborative, respectful, and potentially more effective in nudging patients toward healthier choices—choices they make for their own reasons.

Foundational Insights

- Motivational Interviewing is grounded in a specific "Spirit" (PACE) which is more important than the techniques alone.

- **Partnership** means collaborating with patients as equals, recognizing their expertise in their own lives.

- **Acceptance** involves valuing the patient (absolute worth), understanding their perspective (accurate empathy), respecting their choices (autonomy), and acknowledging their strengths (affirmation).

- **Compassion** is the genuine commitment to the patient's well-being that drives the interaction.

- **Evocation** focuses on drawing out the patient's *own* reasons and ideas for change, rather than imposing external ones.

- Four guiding principles flow from the spirit: **Expressing Empathy** (demonstrating understanding), **Developing Discrepancy** (helping patients see the gap between behavior and goals), **Rolling with Resistance** (avoiding arguments), and **Supporting Self-Efficacy** (building confidence).

- Applying the MI spirit and principles transforms even brief nursing interactions, making them more respectful, collaborative, and effective.

Understanding the MI mindset—the spirit and principles—is the essential first step. It provides the "why" and the "how" of our overall approach. Now, let's equip ourselves with the specific tools that bring this spirit to life in conversation. Chapter 2 introduces the core MI skills known as OARS, the practical building blocks for engaging patients effectively.

Chapter 2: Your MI Toolkit- Mastering the Core Skills (OARS) in Minutes

Having explored the foundational spirit and principles of Motivational Interviewing, we now turn to the practical tools—the specific communication skills that allow you to put that spirit into action. These core skills are often remembered by the acronym **OARS**:

- **O**pen Questions
- **A**ffirmations
- **R**eflections
- **S**ummaries

These are not necessarily new communication techniques—you likely use some form of them already. The power of OARS within MI lies in their **purposeful and skillful application**, guided by the spirit of Partnership, Acceptance, Compassion, and Evocation, and informed by the principles of expressing empathy, developing discrepancy, rolling with resistance, and supporting self-efficacy. Think of OARS as the oars of a boat; used skillfully together, they help you navigate the conversation collaboratively with the patient toward their goals. Master these, even in brief interactions, and you'll find your conversations about change becoming significantly more productive.

The Four Foundational Skills: OARS

Let's examine each skill, focusing on how you can use it efficiently and effectively in your nursing practice.

O: Open Questions - Inviting Exploration

Open questions are those that invite more than a simple "yes" or "no" answer, or a short factual response. They encourage patients to think, elaborate, explore their experiences, and share their perspectives. They typically begin with words like "What," "How," "Tell me about," "Describe," or sometimes "Why" (though "why" can sometimes sound accusatory, so use it thoughtfully). They are the opposite of closed questions, which usually start with "Do," "Did," "Are," "Is," "Will," or "Have," and tend to shut down conversation.

- **Purpose in MI:** To gather information from the patient's perspective, understand their world, elicit their thoughts and feelings about change, and encourage them to talk more (especially about change).
- **Contrast with Closed Questions:**
    - *Closed:* "Did you take your medication this morning?" (Answer: Yes/No)
    - *Open:* "How did it go with taking your medication this morning?" (Invites description, potential barriers, feelings).
    - *Closed:* "Are you worried about the surgery?" (Answer: Yes/No)
    - *Open:* "What are your thoughts or concerns as you think about the upcoming surgery?" (Invites elaboration).
    - *Closed:* "Do you want to quit smoking?" (Answer: Yes/No/Maybe)

- *Open:* "What role does smoking play in your life right now?" or "What are the things you like, and the things you don't like, about smoking?" (Invites exploration of ambivalence).
- **Nursing Focus: Quick-Use Examples:**
  - **During Assessment:**
    - "Tell me about what brought you in today." (Instead of listing symptoms)
    - "How has your [condition, e.g., breathing, pain] been since your last visit?"
    - "What does a typical day look like for you regarding [behavior, e.g., meals, activity]?"
  - **During Patient Education:**
    - "After hearing that information about the medication, what questions or thoughts come to mind?" (Instead of "Do you have any questions?")
    - "How might this new dietary suggestion fit into your daily routine?"
    - "What challenges do you foresee in trying this?"
  - **During Follow-up/Discharge:**
    - "How are things going with the plan we discussed last time?"

- "What support might you need at home to manage this?"
- "Looking ahead, what feels like the most important next step for you regarding your health?"

- **Key Point:** Using open questions shifts the dynamic. You become a curious listener, genuinely interested in the patient's experience, rather than an interrogator filling out a checklist. This fosters partnership and allows the patient's own motivations and concerns to surface. Aim for a balance—you still need closed questions for specific facts, but deliberately incorporating open questions deepens the conversation.

A: Affirmations - Recognizing Strengths and Efforts

Affirmations are statements that recognize and acknowledge a patient's strengths, resources, efforts, positive intentions, or past successes. They are genuine and specific comments that highlight the positive. They are *not* cheerleading ("You can do it!") or generic praise ("Good job!"). Affirmations build rapport, support self-efficacy, and encourage persistence by focusing on what the patient *is* doing or *has* done right, rather than solely on problems.

- **Purpose in MI:** To build patient confidence, counteract discouragement, reinforce positive behaviors or intentions, and strengthen the therapeutic relationship.
- **How to Phrase Them:** Focus on "you" statements that point to specific positive attributes or actions.

- "You were very resourceful in figuring out how to get a ride here today." (Highlights resourcefulness).
- "It took courage to be so honest about how difficult this has been." (Highlights honesty/courage).
- "You've clearly put a lot of thought into this." (Highlights thoughtfulness).
- "You were persistent in calling back to get this appointment scheduled." (Highlights persistence).
- "Even though it was tough, you managed to [positive action, e.g., check your blood sugar twice] yesterday. That shows real effort." (Highlights effort despite difficulty).
- "You're someone who really cares about your family's well-being." (Highlights a core value).

- **Nursing Focus: Finding Opportunities:** Affirmations can be woven into almost any interaction. Listen for opportunities to notice and comment on:
  - **Effort:** "You worked hard to track your food intake this week."
  - **Persistence:** "You kept trying different ways to remember your medication until you found one that worked."
  - **Strengths:** "You have a very organized way of keeping track of your appointments."

- **Values:** "Being independent is clearly very important to you."
- **Coping Skills:** "You handled that stressful situation without resorting to [old behavior], which shows how much you've learned."
- **Honesty:** "I appreciate you sharing that struggle with me."

- **Key Point:** Affirmations must be genuine. Patients can spot false praise easily. Look for authentic positives, even small ones. Affirming effort is often more powerful than affirming outcomes, especially when a patient is struggling. Consistent affirmation helps build the patient's belief in their own ability to succeed.

R: Reflections - Demonstrating Understanding (The Workhorse)

Reflective listening is arguably the most crucial skill in MI. It's the primary way you express empathy and check your understanding. A reflection is not a question, but a statement that reflects back the meaning or feeling of what the patient has said. It shows you are listening, validates their experience, and allows them to hear their own thoughts and feelings voiced back, which can deepen their self-understanding. Good reflections keep the conversation moving and often encourage the patient to elaborate further.

- **Purpose in MI:** To show you are listening and understand, to express empathy, to check your interpretation, to highlight specific aspects of what the patient said (especially change talk or ambivalence), and to guide the conversation gently without directing.

- **Levels of Reflection:**
    - **Simple Reflection:** Repeats or slightly rephrases what the patient said. Confirms you heard them correctly.
        - *Patient:* "I'm just so tired of dealing with this pain every day."
        - *Nurse:* "You're really feeling worn out by the constant pain."
    - **Complex Reflection:** Paraphrases, makes a guess about the underlying meaning or feeling, or reflects implications. These are deeper and often more powerful.
        - *Patient:* "I know I should test my blood sugar, but I hate needles and sometimes I just don't want to know the number."
        - *Nurse (Meaning):* "So the discomfort and maybe fear around the process sometimes outweigh the knowing."
        - *Nurse (Feeling):* "It sounds like you feel quite anxious about the whole procedure and what the results might mean."
    - **Amplified Reflection:** Reflects what the patient said in a slightly exaggerated way (without sarcasm) to encourage them to

perhaps back off an extreme statement or explore the other side. Use with care.

- *Patient:* "There's absolutely no way I can cut down on coffee."
- *Nurse:* "So, coffee is so essential, you can't imagine living without it at all." (This might prompt the patient to say, "Well, maybe not *that* essential...")

  - **Double-Sided Reflection:** Captures both sides of the patient's ambivalence in one statement, often using "and" or "on the one hand... on the other hand..."

    - *Patient:* "I want to exercise more for my health, but I just have zero energy after work."
    - *Nurse:* "On the one hand, getting healthier is important to you, and on the other hand, finding the energy after a long day feels impossible right now."

- **Nursing Focus: Using Reflections Efficiently:**
  - **Keep them concise:** Reflections don't need to be long.
  - **Use a statement tone:** End with your voice going down, not up like a question. (e.g., "You're worried." not "Are you worried?")
  - **Start with stems (optional):** "It sounds like..." "You're feeling..." "So you..." "It seems to you that..."

- **Focus on change talk:** When you hear the patient express desire, ability, reasons, or need for change, reflect it back to emphasize it. ("You really want to be able to play with your kids without getting winded.")

- **Reflect resistance:** Reflecting discord non-judgmentally can de-escalate tension. ("You're not convinced this plan is going to work for you.")

- **Key Point:** Reflections are hypotheses about meaning. If your reflection is slightly off, the patient will usually correct you, which still advances the conversation and understanding. Skillful reflection is the engine of MI—it builds empathy, explores ambivalence, and guides the patient toward their own conclusions.

S: Summaries - Pulling Threads Together

Summaries are essentially extended reflections. They collect pieces of what the patient has said—perhaps feelings, change talk, points of ambivalence, plans—and present them back in a concise package. Summaries show you've been listening attentively, help organize the conversation, reinforce key points (especially change talk), and can be used to shift focus or transition to a new topic or phase (like planning).

- **Purpose in MI:** To demonstrate understanding, structure the conversation, link related ideas, emphasize change talk, highlight ambivalence, check priorities, and transition smoothly.

- **Types of Summaries:**

- **Collecting Summary:** Briefly pulls together several related points the patient has made recently. ("So let me see if I've got this right. You're feeling frustrated with your current weight, you're worried about your blood pressure, and you've been thinking that becoming more active might help with both. Is that about right?")
- **Linking Summary:** Connects something the patient just said with something discussed earlier. ("That desire you just mentioned to have more energy connects back to what you were saying earlier about wanting to keep up with your grandkids.")
- **Transitional Summary:** Wraps up a topic or phase of the conversation and sets the stage for the next step, often ending with an open question. ("Okay, so we've talked quite a bit about the challenges you face with taking medication consistently, and also about your strong desire to stay healthy for your family. Where does this leave you? What are you thinking might be the next step?")

- **Nursing Focus: When to Summarize:**
    - **After exploring a topic:** Before moving on, summarize the key points.
    - **When you feel stuck:** A summary can help refocus the conversation.

- **To highlight change talk:** Gather all the patient's stated reasons/desires for change into one summary.

- **At the end of an encounter:** Summarize key decisions, plans, or understandings. ("So, to recap our conversation, we discussed how managing stress is a big factor for you right now. You decided that trying that 5-minute breathing exercise twice a day feels like a manageable first step, and you'll let me know how it goes at our next check-in. Does that sound accurate?")

- **Key Point:** Good summaries are selective—you don't repeat everything. Focus on the most salient points, particularly those related to motivation and change. Always check for accuracy ("Did I get that right?" "Is there anything I missed?"). Summaries act like signposts, helping both you and the patient see where you've been and where you might be going.

Putting OARS Together: A Brief Example

Let's revisit Nurse Davis and Mr. Chen (Type 2 diabetes, high A1c), but this time Nurse Davis uses OARS guided by the MI spirit.

Nurse Davis: "Mr. Chen, thanks for coming in. We got your lab results back, and your A1c is 9.2 percent today. That's higher than we were aiming for. **What are your thoughts about that number?**" (**Open Question**)

Mr. Chen: (Looks down) "Yeah, it's not good. I guess I haven't been doing great with the diet... or checking my sugars like I should."

Nurse Davis: "**So you're recognizing that things haven't gone exactly as planned regarding your diet and blood sugar checks.**" (**Simple Reflection**) "**It sounds like managing it all has been pretty challenging lately.**" (**Complex Reflection** – guessing at feeling)

Mr. Chen: "It really has. Work has been so stressful, just crazy hours. By the time I get home, I'm exhausted. Grabbing a soda is easy, and checking my sugar feels like one more thing I failed at."

Nurse Davis: "**It takes a lot of effort to manage diabetes, especially when life throws extra stress your way.**" (**Affirmation** of difficulty/struggle) "**And it sounds like you're feeling discouraged, maybe even seeing it as a failure when you can't keep up with it perfectly.**" (**Complex Reflection** – feeling/meaning)

Mr. Chen: "Exactly! Like, what's the point if I mess up anyway?"

Nurse Davis: "**So that feeling of discouragement makes you wonder if the effort is even worthwhile.**" (**Reflection**) "**Tell me a bit more about what makes checking your sugar feel particularly difficult right now?**" (**Open Question**)

Mr. Chen: "Well, besides hating the finger stick, it's just... if the number is high, I feel bad. If it's low, I worry. It's always something."

Nurse Davis: "**You find yourself reacting emotionally to the numbers, feeling bad or worried regardless of the result.**" (**Reflection**) "**And you're also someone who, despite these challenges, continues to come to these appointments** and talk honestly about what's going on, which shows you haven't given up." (**Affirmation** of persistence/honesty)

Mr. Chen: "Well, yeah. I don't *want* to get sick. My dad had terrible problems with his diabetes."

Nurse Davis: "**So avoiding those kinds of problems your dad faced is a strong motivator for you.**" (**Reflection** – highlighting change talk/reason) "**Okay, let me see if I'm following you. On one hand, managing the daily tasks like checking sugar and diet feels really burdensome and discouraging right now, especially with work stress. On the other hand, you have a powerful reason—not wanting to experience the serious complications your dad did—that keeps you engaged in trying to manage your health. Is that capturing it?**" (**Summary** – double-sided, linking, transitional)

Mr. Chen: "Yeah, that's pretty much it."

Nurse Davis: "**Given that, what feels like a possible next step for you, even a small one, in managing things right now?**" (**Open Question** – inviting collaboration/planning)

Notice how OARS skills, guided by empathy and partnership, create a very different conversation. Nurse Davis isn't lecturing; she's listening, understanding, affirming, and gently guiding Mr. Chen to explore his own situation and motivation. This is the practical application of the MI spirit, facilitated by these core communication tools.

Practical Tools Summary

- The OARS skills (Open Questions, Affirmations, Reflections, Summaries) are the core communication tools of MI.

- **Open Questions** invite exploration and detailed responses, fostering partnership (e.g., "How...?" "What...?" "Tell me about...").

- **Affirmations** recognize patient strengths, efforts, and positive intentions, building self-efficacy (e.g., "You showed real determination by...").

- **Reflections** demonstrate empathy and understanding by stating back the meaning or feeling of what the patient said (Simple, Complex, Amplified, Double-Sided). They are central to MI.

- **Summaries** pull together key points, organize the conversation, emphasize change talk, and facilitate transitions (Collecting, Linking, Transitional).

- Using OARS purposefully and skillfully, guided by the MI spirit, transforms routine nursing interactions into opportunities for collaborative exploration of change.

- These skills can be integrated efficiently into brief encounters during assessments, education, and follow-up.

Mastering the OARS skills provides you with the essential toolkit for Motivational Interviewing. Now that you have the tools, the next step is learning how to listen specifically for the sparks of motivation within the conversation—what we call "change talk." Chapter 3 will focus on how to recognize these crucial patient statements and how to respond in ways that gently fan those sparks into flames of change.

Chapter 3: Listening for Change- Recognizing and Responding to Change Talk

You've embraced the MI spirit – that foundation of Partnership, Acceptance, Compassion, and Evocation. You're becoming more comfortable with your OARS toolkit – Open questions, Affirmations, Reflections, and Summaries. Now, we tune our ears to something specific. In any conversation about behavior change, people express different kinds of speech. Some statements lean toward keeping things the same, while others lean toward making a change. Motivational Interviewing has a particular interest in the latter. This patient speech that favors movement toward a particular change goal is called **change talk**. Learning to recognize, elicit, and respond effectively to change talk is central to guiding patients toward healthier behaviors. It's like panning for gold – you're listening for those valuable nuggets of motivation amidst the stream of conversation.

What is Change Talk Hearing the patients arguments for change

Simply put, **change talk is any self-expressed language from the patient that is an argument for change**. It's not you telling them why they should change; it's them telling *you* (and themselves) why they might want to, need to, or are able to change. It's the manifestation of the "evocation" part of the MI spirit. You're listening for the patient's own voice articulating reasons, desires, abilities, needs, or commitment related to a specific behavior change.

Why is this so important? Decades of research have shown a clear link: **the more someone voices their own arguments for change, the more likely they are to actually make that change**. It's predictive. When you hear change talk, you're hearing the seeds of potential action. Your job, using MI skills, is to help cultivate those seeds. Conversely, if the conversation is dominated by "sustain talk"—the arguments for *not* changing—actual change becomes less likely. Therefore, skillfully navigating the conversation to elicit and reinforce change talk is a key nursing function when addressing health behaviors.

The DARN-CAT Mnemonic Recognizing Kinds of Change Talk

To help identify the different flavors of change talk, the mnemonic **DARN-CAT** is incredibly useful. It categorizes change talk into two groups: preparatory change talk (DARN) and mobilizing change talk (CAT).

Preparatory Change Talk (DARN): Setting the Stage

This type of talk expresses motivation but doesn't necessarily signal immediate action. It indicates the patient is *thinking* about change, exploring the possibility.

1. **D**esire: Statements about wanting, wishing, or liking the idea of change.
    - "I **want** to feel healthier."
    - "I **wish** I could control my temper better."
    - "I'd **like** to be able to play with my grandkids without getting short of breath."
    - "It **would be nice** to not rely on cigarettes."

2. **A**bility: Statements expressing perceived capability or confidence in making the change. Often includes words like "can," "could," "able," "possible."
    - "*I **could probably** walk for 10 minutes each day.*"
    - "*I **think I can** manage taking the pills twice a day instead of three times.*"
    - "*I was **able** to quit drinking sodas for a month last year.*"
    - "*Maybe it's **possible** for me to try that breathing exercise.*"

3. **R**eason: Statements outlining specific reasons, benefits, or advantages of making the change. Often answers the "why" question.
    - "*If I lost some weight, my joints **would probably hurt less**.*"
    - "*Quitting smoking **would save me a lot of money**.*"
    - "*Taking my medication regularly **might prevent me from having another flare-up**.*"
    - "*My family **would be happier** if I wasn't drinking so much.*"

4. **N**eed: Statements expressing an urgency or necessity for change. Often uses words like "need," "must," "have to," "got to," "important."
    - "*I **need** to do something about my stress levels.*"

- "I really **must** get my blood pressure under control."
- "It's **important** for me to manage my diet better now."
- "I've **got to** stop missing my appointments."

Mobilizing Change Talk (CAT): Signaling Movement

This type of talk signals the patient is moving beyond just thinking about change and is closer to taking action. It often follows preparatory talk.

5. **C**ommitment: Statements expressing a specific intention, decision, or promise to act. Uses words like "will," "intend to," "promise," "going to," "ready to." This is the strongest form of change talk.

    - "I **will** start walking tomorrow morning."
    - "I **intend to** fill that prescription today."
    - "I **promise** myself I won't smoke in the house anymore."
    - "I'm **going to** try packing my lunch instead of buying fast food."
    - "I'm **ready to** set a quit date."

6. **A**ctivation: Statements indicating movement toward action, without quite being a full commitment. Uses words like "willing to," "prepared to," "considering."

    - "I'm **willing to** try cutting back on sugary drinks."

- "I'm **prepared to** check my blood sugar at least once a day."
- "I've been **considering** joining that support group."
- "Maybe I **could** start by just leaving my cigarettes at home when I go out."

7. **T**aking **S**teps: Statements reporting on actions already taken toward the change goal.

    - "I **bought** some nicotine patches yesterday."
    - "I **looked up** the schedule for the exercise class at the community center."
    - "I actually **walked** around the block twice this morning."
    - "I **threw out** all the junk food in my pantry."

Recognizing these different types helps you gauge where the patient is in their process and tailor your responses accordingly. DARN talk is good; CAT talk is even better, as it more strongly predicts action.

How to Elicit Change Talk Using OARS strategically

You don't just passively wait for change talk to appear; you actively use your OARS skills to invite it. Here's how:

1. **Ask Evocative Open Questions:** Frame questions specifically designed to elicit DARN-CAT statements.

    - *Desire:* "What do you **hope** to get out of making this change?" "How would you **like** things to be different?"

- *Ability:* "If you did decide to make this change, how **could** you do it?" "What **might be possible** for you?" "How confident are you that you **could** manage that?" (Use scaling questions: "On a scale of 0 to 10, where 0 is not at all confident and 10 is very confident, how confident are you that you could [take a specific step]?") Follow up with: "Why did you choose a [number] and not a [lower number]?" (This often elicits ability talk).

- *Reasons:* "What are some of the **advantages** you see in [making the change]?" "What's the **downside** of how things are now?" "What **worries** you about your current [behavior]?"

- *Need:* "How **important** is it for you to [make the change] right now?" "What do you think **needs** to happen?"

- *Commitment/Activation/Taking Steps:* "What do you think you **will** do?" "What are you **willing** to try?" "What steps have you **already considered** or **taken**?" "What seems like the **next step**?"

2. **Use Reflections Strategically:** Reflect any change talk you hear clearly and concisely. This reinforces it and encourages the patient to elaborate. Especially reflect DARN components.

    - *Patient:* "I guess my breathing would be better if I stopped smoking." (Reason)
    - *Nurse:* "You think your breathing might improve." (Simple Reflection) or "So, one clear

53

benefit for you would be easier breathing." (Complex Reflection)

3. **Use Affirmations When You Hear Change Talk:** Affirm the patient's efforts, intentions, or awareness related to change.
    - *Patient:* "I managed to go for a walk three times this week." (Taking Steps)
    - *Nurse:* "That took real commitment to fit those walks into your schedule." (Affirmation)

4. **Use Summaries to Collect Change Talk:** Gather multiple change talk statements together to reinforce the patient's own motivation.
    - *Nurse:* "So, if I'm hearing you correctly, you're saying you **want** to have more energy (Desire), you think you **could** probably start with short walks (Ability), especially because you know it **would help** your blood sugar (Reason) and it feels **important** to be healthier for your kids (Need). That's a lot of good reasons pointing toward making a change." (Collecting Summary emphasizing DARN)

Responding to Change Talk Reinforcing the positive EARS

When a patient offers change talk, it's a critical moment. How you respond can either encourage further exploration or shut it down. The goal is to reinforce the change talk. A helpful mnemonic for responding effectively is **EARS**:

- **E**laborate: Ask for more details, examples, or the "why" behind the change talk. Use open questions.

- "Tell me more about that."
- "In what ways would that be helpful?"
- "What does that look like for you?"
- "Give me an example."

- **A**ffirm: Directly affirm the change talk comment or the underlying intention/strength.
  - "That sounds like a great idea."
  - "It's clear you've given this some thought."
  - "That shows real commitment to your health."

- **R**eflect: Reflect the change talk back to the patient, perhaps emphasizing it slightly.
  - "So, making that change is becoming more important to you."
  - "You really want things to be different."
  - "You're starting to think you could actually do this."

- **S**ummarize: Collect several change talk statements together. (As described above).

Using EARS helps the patient hear their own arguments for change amplified and validated, strengthening their motivation.

Case Study: Maria - Community Health Nurse and Change Talk

Sarah, a community health nurse, is visiting Maria, a 35-year-old mother of two young children who smokes about a pack a day. Maria has expressed wanting to quit "someday" but feels overwhelmed.

Sarah: "Maria, we've talked about smoking before. What are your thoughts about it today?" (**Open Question**)

Maria: "Ugh, I know I should quit. It costs so much money, and sometimes I worry about getting sick like my aunt did... she had lung cancer. But honestly, with the kids and work, it's my only break. It's how I cope."

Sarah: "So on one hand, the cost and the worry about your health—especially thinking about your aunt—are significant downsides for you." (**Reflection** - Reasons/Need). "And on the other hand, smoking feels like a really essential coping tool right now, maybe your main way to get a moment to yourself." (**Reflection** - Sustain talk/function of behavior). "That sounds like a tough spot to be in." (**Reflection** - Empathy).

Maria: "It really is. I **wish** I didn't need it." (**Desire**)

Sarah: "**You wish things were different, that you didn't feel that need for cigarettes.**" (**Reflection** - Desire). "**Tell me more about that wish.** What would be better if you didn't need them?" (**Elaborate** - Asking for Reasons)

Maria: "Well, I'd save money, obviously. Maybe almost $300 a month! And I wouldn't worry so much about getting cancer. And maybe I'd have more energy... sometimes I feel sluggish." (**Reasons**)

Sarah: "**Saving that much money each month would make a difference, and you'd feel less worried about your health and maybe have more energy too.** Those are some powerful reasons." (**Summary** of Reasons, **Affirmation**).

Maria: "Yeah... I tried quitting once before, cold turkey. Lasted three days. It was awful."

Sarah: "**You've tried quitting before, which shows it's something you've seriously considered and have experience with, even though that attempt was really difficult.**" (**Affirmation** of effort/past attempt, **Reflection**). "**What did you learn from that experience?**" (**Open Question** - exploring Ability/past learning)

Maria: "That cold turkey is probably not for me! And that the cravings were worst in the morning and after meals."

Sarah: "**So you learned something really useful about your patterns and maybe about needing a different approach than cold turkey.** That's valuable information." (**Reflection**, **Affirmation** of learning). "**Given that, what might be a small step you could consider now, even if it's not full quitting?**" (**Open Question** - exploring Ability/Activation)

Maria: "Hmm. Maybe... maybe I **could** try not smoking in the car? The kids complain about the smell anyway." (**Ability**, hinting at Reason - kids complaining)

Sarah: "**So one possibility you're considering is making the car a smoke-free zone.**" (**Reflection** - Activation/Ability). "**That sounds like a concrete step.** How confident are you that you **could** do that for, say, the next week?" (**Affirmation**, **Open Question** - exploring confidence/Ability)

In this exchange, Sarah skillfully uses OARS to navigate Maria's ambivalence, listens carefully for DARN elements (Desire, Reason, Ability), reflects and affirms them (EARS), and gently guides Maria toward considering a specific, manageable step (Activation/Ability). She doesn't push; she evokes and reinforces Maria's own change talk.

Distinguishing Change Talk from Sustain Talk Arguments for not changing

Just as important as recognizing change talk is recognizing its counterpart: **sustain talk**. This is any patient speech that argues *against* change, favoring the status quo. It includes reasons *not* to change, perceived inability to change, lack of desire or need for change, or commitment *not* to change.

- **Examples of Sustain Talk:**
    - "*I* don't **want** to give up my favorite foods." (Desire for status quo)
    - "*I* **can't** imagine fitting exercise into my day." (Perceived inability to change)
    - "*Smoking* **relaxes** *me; I need that.*" (Reason to maintain status quo)
    - "*It's* **not that important** *for me to lose weight right now.*" (Lack of need for change)
    - "*I* **won't** *take that medication; the side effects sound terrible.*" (Commitment against change)

It's normal for patients to express both change talk and sustain talk, often in the same breath—that's ambivalence! Your goal isn't to shut down sustain talk directly (which often leads to resistance), but to acknowledge it with reflective listening ("So, that relaxation is something you really value about smoking") and then gently guide the conversation back toward exploring the change side ("And what are some of the things you *don't* like about smoking?"). You want to selectively reinforce the change talk using EARS, giving it more airtime and emphasis in the conversation.

Nursing Focus Identifying change talk amidst routine conversations

Change talk doesn't always arrive neatly packaged. It often emerges subtly within routine nursing interactions. Your task is to develop "MI ears" to catch it.

- **During Medication Review:**
    - *Patient:* "This new pill makes me feel a bit fuzzy in the morning, but I guess **it's better than having another stroke**." (Sustain talk about side effect + **Reason** for change/adherence).
    - *Nurse Response (Reflecting change talk):* "**Preventing another stroke is clearly a major priority for you.**"
- **Discussing Diet:**
    - *Patient:* "My wife keeps telling me to eat more vegetables. I don't love them, but maybe **I'd feel less sluggish if I tried**." (Sustain talk about preference + **Ability/Reason** for change).
    - *Nurse Response (Elaborating on change talk):* "**Tell me more about feeling less sluggish. How would that make a difference for you?**"
- **Talking About Activity:**
    - *Patient:* "My knee hurts when I walk too much, so I mostly sit. **I wish I could be more active**

like I used to be though." (Sustain talk about barrier + **Desire** for change).

- *Nurse Response (Reflecting change talk):* "**You really miss being more active.**"

- **Checking Blood Sugar Logs:**

  - *Patient:* "I only checked twice yesterday, I know I should do it more. **I'm going to try harder this week.**" (Acknowledges falling short + **Commitment**).

  - *Nurse Response (Affirming change talk):* "**Setting that intention to try harder this week shows your commitment to managing this.**"

By actively listening for DARN-CAT language within these everyday conversations and responding with EARS (Elaborate, Affirm, Reflect, Summarize), you significantly increase the chances of reinforcing the patient's natural movement toward positive health behavior change.

Tuning In Key Points

- **Change Talk** is any patient statement favoring movement toward change; it predicts actual behavior change.

- **Sustain Talk** is any patient statement favoring the status quo. Ambivalence involves both.

- The **DARN-CAT** mnemonic helps categorize change talk:

- **Preparatory (DARN):** Desire, Ability, Reason, Need.
- **Mobilizing (CAT):** Commitment, Activation, Taking Steps.

- Use **OARS strategically** (especially Open Questions and Reflections) to elicit change talk.
- Respond to change talk using **EARS** to reinforce it: Elaborate, Affirm, Reflect, Summarize.
- Develop "MI ears" to identify change talk subtly emerging in routine nursing interactions about medications, diet, activity, etc.
- Acknowledge sustain talk with reflections, but selectively reinforce change talk.

Listening for change talk is essential, but conversations aren't always smooth. Often, you'll encounter the other side of the coin: sustain talk and moments where the conversation feels stuck or tense—what MI calls discord. Chapter 4 focuses on understanding this natural ambivalence and discord, and provides strategies for "dancing" with it effectively, avoiding arguments and keeping the door open for change.

Chapter 4: Dancing with Discord- Navigating Ambivalence and Rolling with Resistance

We've focused on listening for and encouraging the positive side of motivation—change talk. But as any nurse knows, conversations about health behavior don't always flow smoothly toward commitment. More often than not, you encounter **ambivalence**: that state of feeling pulled in two directions simultaneously. *"I want to quit smoking, but I enjoy it." "I know I need to take this medication, but I hate the side effects."* Alongside ambivalence, you might encounter moments where the interaction feels tense, where the patient seems argumentative, dismissive, or withdrawn. In MI, we call this **discord**, signaling a friction *in the relationship*, not necessarily a fixed characteristic of the patient. Understanding how to navigate both ambivalence and discord without falling into common communication traps is essential for maintaining a collaborative partnership. This chapter is about learning the steps to "dance" with these challenging moments, rather than wrestling against them.

Understanding Ambivalence Its normal to feel two ways about change

First and foremost, **ambivalence is normal**. It's a natural human state when considering any significant change. Change involves giving something up (a habit, a comfort, the status quo) to gain something else (better health, more energy, fewer risks). Feeling torn between the familiar and the potentially better is completely expected.

Think about a change *you've* considered—starting an exercise routine, eating healthier, learning a new skill. Didn't you have reasons *for* doing it and reasons *for not* doing it? Weren't there perceived benefits and perceived costs or difficulties? Patients are no different. When they express ambivalence ("I know I should, but..."), they aren't necessarily being difficult or unmotivated. They are simply expressing the internal tug-of-war that precedes change.

Your role in MI is not to immediately try to resolve the ambivalence *for* them by telling them why the "pro-change" side is right. Instead, your role is to **help them explore both sides of their ambivalence openly and without judgment**. Using reflections, especially double-sided reflections, is key here.

- *Patient:* "I know exercising would help my blood sugar, but I honestly just don't have the time."
- *Nurse (Double-sided reflection):* "So on one hand, you see a clear health benefit to exercising in terms of your blood sugar, and on the other hand, fitting it into your current schedule feels completely impossible."

By reflecting both sides, you show you understand their dilemma, validate their conflict, and allow them to hear their own ambivalence voiced back. This process of exploration is often what helps individuals eventually tip the balance toward change for themselves. Trying to force the issue usually just strengthens their attachment to the "status quo" side of the argument.

Recognizing Sustain Talk and Discord Resistance is often a signal about our approach

As patients explore ambivalence, you will naturally hear **sustain talk**—the arguments for *not* changing. As we discussed in the last chapter, this includes statements about desiring the status quo, feeling unable to change, seeing reasons not to change, or feeling no need to change. Examples: "I like my salty snacks," "I've tried quitting before and failed," "This medication costs too much," "My breathing isn't *that* bad."

It's how you *respond* to sustain talk that matters. If you directly challenge it, argue against it, or dismiss it, you often provoke **discord**. Discord used to be called "resistance," but MI shifted the language to emphasize that it's not solely a patient characteristic; it often arises from the *interaction*. Discord is like friction or static in the communication channel. It signals a breakdown in the collaborative relationship.

Signs of Discord:

- **Arguing/Challenging:** The patient directly contests your accuracy, expertise, or integrity ("That's not true," "You don't understand").

- **Interrupting:** The patient talks over you, often defensively.

- **Discounting/Ignoring:** The patient dismisses your concerns or suggestions ("That won't work for me," "This isn't a big deal"). They might change the subject abruptly or ignore you.

- **Hostility/Negative Emotional Tone:** The patient expresses irritation, anger, sarcasm, or impatience through words or body language (sighing, eye-rolling, crossed arms).
- **Appearing Passive:** While seeming to agree ("Yeah, yeah, okay"), their body language or lack of engagement suggests they are just placating you to end the conversation.

When you sense discord, it's a cue to **change your approach**. It's often a signal that you might have inadvertently slipped into the "righting reflex," pushed too hard, offered unsolicited advice, misunderstood the patient, or failed to adequately express empathy or partnership. Blaming the patient for being "resistant" is unproductive. Instead, ask yourself: "What am I doing that's contributing to this friction, and how can I shift back to a more collaborative stance?"

Avoiding the Communication Traps The Righting Reflex questioning traps premature focus

Several common communication patterns reliably generate discord and hinder progress. Becoming aware of these traps is the first step to avoiding them.

1. **The Righting Reflex:** This is the most common trap for helpers. It's our natural desire to fix problems, give advice, and make things right for the patient. When a patient expresses a problem or ambivalence, we jump in with solutions, warnings, or persuasion. *"You really need to..." "You should..." "Have you tried...?"* While well-intentioned, this often makes the patient feel unheard, misunderstood, or pressured,

prompting them to defend their position (i.e., argue *for* the status quo). You take the "pro-change" side, forcing them into the "anti-change" side.

2. **Question-Answer Trap (Interrogation):** Asking too many closed questions in a row can make the interaction feel like an interrogation. The nurse asks, the patient gives a short answer, the nurse asks another question... This puts the patient in a passive role and limits exploration. It lacks the flow and collaboration of an MI conversation rich with reflections.

3. **Taking Sides/Arguing:** Directly disagreeing with a patient or arguing about the benefits of change ("No, quitting smoking isn't *that* hard if you really try!") immediately creates an adversarial dynamic. You cannot win this argument; you only solidify their opposition.

4. **Expert Trap:** Presenting yourself as the sole authority who has all the answers and simply needs to educate the passive patient. This undermines partnership and the patient's sense of autonomy and expertise in their own life.

5. **Labeling Trap:** Applying diagnostic labels or character judgments ("You're in denial," "You're being non-compliant," "You seem unmotivated"). Labels can feel stigmatizing and often provoke defensiveness. MI focuses on behaviors and perspectives, not fixed labels.

6. **Premature Focus Trap:** Trying to focus on a specific behavior change (e.g., diet) before establishing

rapport, understanding the patient's perspective, or exploring their *own* priorities. If the patient isn't concerned about their diet, but you keep pushing it, discord is likely. You need to find common ground first.

7. **Blaming Trap:** Implying the patient is at fault for their problems ("Well, if you hadn't eaten all that cake, your blood sugar wouldn't be so high"). Blame and shame rarely motivate positive change; they usually lead to withdrawal or defensiveness.

Avoiding these traps requires conscious effort and adherence to the MI spirit and skills—listening more than talking, reflecting rather than questioning excessively, asking permission before advising, and always maintaining a stance of partnership and respect.

Strategies for Rolling with Resistance Dancing with Discord

When discord arises despite your best efforts, MI offers specific strategies not to *fight* it, but to "roll with it"—like a judo master using the opponent's momentum rather than directly opposing their force. These techniques aim to defuse tension, acknowledge the patient's perspective, and gently redirect the conversation back toward collaboration.

1. **Simple Reflection:** This is often the first and best response. Simply reflect the content or feeling of the patient's sustain talk or discordant statement without judgment. This shows you heard them and accepts their perspective *as their perspective*.
    - *Patient:* "This is pointless! Nothing ever works for me."

- *Nurse:* "It feels like you've tried everything and nothing has made a difference, leaving you feeling pretty hopeless right now."
- *Patient:* "You don't understand how hard it is!"
- *Nurse:* "It seems like I'm not fully grasping the challenges you're facing."

2. **Shifting Focus:** You can sometimes defuse discord by redirecting the conversation away from the sticking point, at least temporarily. Acknowledge the issue, then gently change direction.
    - *Patient:* "There's no way I'm taking that medication with those side effects!"
    - *Nurse:* "Those potential side effects sound really concerning to you (Reflection). We can certainly talk more about that. For a moment, could we perhaps shift gears and talk about what's been going well with managing your [condition] lately?" (Shifting Focus).

3. **Reframing:** Offer a different meaning or interpretation of what the patient is saying. A reframe acknowledges the validity of their observation but casts it in a new light that might be more constructive or open to solutions.
    - *Patient:* "I failed completely at sticking to the diet last week."
    - *Nurse:* "So, last week didn't go as you planned, and it sounds like you learned some things about what makes sticking to the diet difficult

for you right now." (Reframing "failure" as a "learning experience").

- *Patient:* "My family keeps nagging me about my smoking."
- *Nurse:* "It sounds like they care about you and are worried about your health, even if the way they express it feels like nagging." (Reframing "nagging" as "caring/concern").

4. **Emphasizing Personal Choice and Control (Affirming Autonomy):** When patients feel pushed, explicitly affirming their autonomy can reduce discord. Reminding them that ultimately, the decision is theirs, can paradoxically make them *less* resistant to considering change.

    - *Patient:* "Everyone keeps telling me I have to quit drinking coffee!"
    - *Nurse:* "It sounds like you're feeling pressured from a lot of directions. I want to be clear – what you decide to do about your coffee intake is entirely up to you. My role is just to help you think through the options if you're interested."
    - *Patient:* (After nurse explains benefits of therapy) "I'm still not sure I want to go."
    - *Nurse:* "And that's absolutely your call to make. You're the expert on what feels right for you."

5. **Agreeing with a Twist (Reflection + Reframe):** Reflect part of what the patient says, and then add a slight reframe that points toward change.

- *Patient:* "I know I should exercise, but I just hate feeling breathless."
- *Nurse:* "You really dislike that feeling of breathlessness (Reflection), *and* you're looking for ways to manage your health that feel more comfortable for you (Reframe)."

Case Study: David - Handling Medication Reluctance in Mental Health

Mark, a mental health nurse, is talking with David, a young man diagnosed with schizophrenia who has been reluctant to consistently take his prescribed antipsychotic medication due to weight gain.

Mark: "David, how have things been going with taking the medication since we last talked?" (**Open Question**)

David: "It's stupid. I hate it. It makes me fat and sleepy." (**Sustain Talk/Discord**)

Mark (Option 1 - Righting Reflex - Avoid this): "David, you know how important this medication is for preventing relapse. The weight gain is manageable if you watch your diet..." (This likely leads to more argument).

Mark (Option 2 - Rolling with Discord): "**It sounds like you really dislike the medication because of the side effects, particularly the weight gain and drowsiness, and maybe you even feel it's pointless.**" (**Simple/Complex Reflection** acknowledging sustain talk and feeling).

David: "Yeah! What's the point of not hearing voices if I feel like a zombie and none of my clothes fit?"

Mark: "**So from your perspective, the trade-off feels terrible right now – the side effects seem worse than the symptoms they're treating.**" (**Complex Reflection**). "**It's understandable why you'd feel reluctant to take something that makes you feel that way.**" (**Empathy/Acceptance**).

David: (Slightly less tense) "Well, yeah."

Mark: "**You know, it takes courage to talk so openly about these frustrations.**" (**Affirmation**). "**And ultimately, deciding what you do about medication is your choice.**" (**Emphasizing Personal Choice**). "**I'm wondering, on the other side of things, what, if anything, have you noticed that's been better when you** *have* **taken the medication regularly in the past?**" (**Shifting Focus slightly back to potential benefits/Evocation**)

David: "Well… I guess I wasn't arguing with my mom as much. And I could focus a bit better on my video games." (**Change Talk - Reasons**)

Mark: "**So, when you were taking it, things were calmer with your mom, and your concentration improved for things you enjoy.**" (**Reflection** of change talk). "**Okay, so we have this situation where the medication helps with focus and family relationships, but the side effects like weight gain and drowsiness are a major problem for you. What are your thoughts on how we might navigate this dilemma?**" (**Summary** of ambivalence, **Open Question** inviting collaboration).

By reflecting David's frustration, affirming his honesty, emphasizing his autonomy, and gently exploring both sides of the ambivalence, Mark avoids an argument and keeps the conversation collaborative. He "rolls with" the discord instead of pushing against it, creating space for David to potentially consider options or compromises later (like discussing alternative medications, dosage adjustments, or strategies to manage side effects).

Nursing Focus De-escalating tense conversations handling medication reluctance addressing missed appointments without blame

The strategies for rolling with discord are directly applicable to common nursing challenges:

- **De-escalating Tense Conversations:** When a patient is angry or upset, start with reflective listening. Show you are trying to understand their frustration ("It sounds incredibly frustrating that you had to wait so long," "You're feeling angry because you feel like no one is listening"). Avoid getting defensive or matching their tone. Emphasize partnership ("Let's see how we might figure this out together").

- **Handling Medication Reluctance:** Avoid the righting reflex. Explore their concerns using open questions ("What worries you most about taking this?"). Reflect their reasons for not wanting to take it ("So the potential side effects sound quite daunting"). Affirm their autonomy ("It's your decision"). Explore ambivalence ("What are the things you *don't* like about *not* taking it?"). If appropriate, use Elicit-Provide-Elicit (Chapter 5) to share information about risks/benefits/alternatives *after* understanding their perspective.

- **Addressing Missed Appointments Without Blame:** Instead of "You missed your appointment again!", try: "I noticed we missed you at your last appointment. How have things been going?" (Open Question, non-blaming). Or reflect potential difficulty: "It can sometimes be really challenging juggling schedules and getting to appointments." Explore barriers collaboratively: "What gets in the way of making it to your appointments sometimes?" Focus on solutions together: "How could we make scheduling work better for you?"

The key is shifting from seeing resistance as patient defiance to seeing discord as a signal to adjust *your* approach back toward partnership, empathy, and respect for autonomy.

Navigating Choppy Waters Key Insights

- **Ambivalence** (feeling two ways about change) is normal and should be explored, not immediately resolved by the nurse.

- **Sustain Talk** (arguments for staying the same) is a natural part of ambivalence.

- **Discord** (arguing, interrupting, hostility, ignoring) signals friction in the nurse-patient relationship, often prompted by the nurse's approach (e.g., the righting reflex).

- Avoid common **Communication Traps** like the Righting Reflex, Interrogation, Arguing, Expert Trap, Labeling, Premature Focus, and Blaming.

- When discord arises, **"Roll With It"** instead of fighting against it.

- Key strategies include **Simple Reflection, Shifting Focus, Reframing,** and **Emphasizing Personal Choice and Control.**

- These strategies are effective for de-escalating tense conversations, addressing medication reluctance non-confrontationally, and discussing missed appointments without blame.

- View discord as a signal to adjust *your* communication back toward the MI spirit.

We've learned how to listen for change talk and how to navigate the inevitable ambivalence and discord that arise in conversations about change. But nursing involves more than just listening and reflecting; a significant part of your role is providing information and education. How do you do that in a way that aligns with the MI spirit, respects patient autonomy, and avoids triggering discord? Chapter 5 introduces the Elicit-Provide-Elicit framework, a method for sharing information effectively and collaboratively.

Chapter 5: Sharing Information Effectively-The Elicit-Provide-Elicit (EPE) Method

So far, we've concentrated heavily on the listening side of Motivational Interviewing—understanding the spirit, using OARS skills, tuning into change talk, and navigating ambivalence and discord. This emphasis is crucial because MI fundamentally shifts the focus from the expert *telling* to the patient *exploring*. However, let's be realistic: as a nurse, providing information, education, and clinical advice is a core part of your professional responsibility. Patients need information about their conditions, treatment options, medication side effects, self-management techniques, and potential health risks. The question isn't *if* you provide information, but *how* you provide it in a way that is consistent with the collaborative, patient-centered spirit of MI. Simply dumping information onto a patient often triggers that "righting reflex" in reverse—they feel lectured, overwhelmed, or resistant. The **Elicit-Provide-Elicit (EPE)** method offers a structured yet flexible way to share information respectfully and effectively, increasing the chances that the patient will actually hear, understand, and consider it.

The Nurses Role as Educator Giving information MI-style

Your role as an educator is undeniable. Patients rely on your knowledge and expertise. Traditional health education often follows a simple model: Assess knowledge gap -> Provide information to fill gap -> Expect behavior change. While straightforward, this often fails because it neglects the patient's own perspective, priorities, readiness, and potential ambivalence. It assumes information alone drives change.

MI-style information exchange, embodied by EPE, approaches education differently:

- It **starts with the patient's perspective**. What do they already know? What do *they* want to know? What are *their* concerns?
- It **asks permission** before offering information, respecting their autonomy.
- It delivers information **clearly, concisely, and neutrally**, avoiding jargon and persuasive language.
- It immediately **checks back** with the patient to understand their reaction, interpretation, and takeaway.
- It places the information within the context of the patient's own goals and values.

This approach transforms information sharing from a one-way lecture into a collaborative dialogue. It ensures the information provided is relevant, timely, and tailored to the individual patient's needs and readiness.

Moving Beyond the Information Dump

We've all seen—and perhaps been guilty of—the "information dump." A patient is newly diagnosed, and we provide a mountain of pamphlets, detailed explanations of pathophysiology, lists of do's and don'ts, and warnings about complications. While well-intentioned, this often results in:

- **Information Overload:** The patient can't possibly absorb or retain everything.

- **Increased Anxiety:** Too much information, especially about risks, can be overwhelming.
- **Passive Reception:** The patient tunes out or nods along without truly engaging.
- **Discord:** If the information feels like a lecture or contradicts the patient's beliefs, it can trigger resistance.
- **Missed Opportunities:** We might spend time explaining things the patient already knows or isn't interested in, while missing what they *actually* want or need to understand.

The EPE method provides a structured alternative that avoids these pitfalls by breaking the process down into manageable, interactive steps.

The EPE Framework A Collaborative Approach

Elicit-Provide-Elicit is a simple, three-step framework:[14]

Step 1: Elicit - Ask what the patient already knows or wants to know. Ask permission.

Before you offer any information, find out what's already on the patient's mind. This serves several purposes: it helps you tailor your information, avoids telling them things they already know, shows respect for their existing knowledge, and gives them control over the flow of information. A key part of this step is explicitly asking permission to share information.

- **Elicit Existing Knowledge/Interest:**
    - "What do you already know about managing high blood pressure?"

- "What have you heard about this medication?"
- "When you think about your diabetes, what aspects are you most curious or concerned about right now?"
- "We have a few different options we could discuss for managing this. What are your initial thoughts or questions about them?"

- **Ask Permission:** This simple step powerfully affirms autonomy.
    - "Would you be interested in hearing a bit about how this medication works?"
    - "I have some information about ways to manage those side effects. Would now be a good time to talk about that?"
    - "Are you open to discussing the connection between smoking and your breathing?"
    - "The lab results show a change we need to discuss. Is now okay to go over what that might mean?"

- **What if they say no?** Respect their decision. You might say, "Okay, perhaps another time. What would be most helpful to discuss right now?" or gently explore the reason, "What makes you hesitant to talk about that now?" Often, simply respecting the "no" makes them more open later.

This initial "Elicit" phase sets the stage for a collaborative exchange. You're finding out where they are starting from and ensuring they are open to receiving information.

Step 2: Provide - Offer information clearly concisely neutrally

Once you have permission and understand the patient's starting point, provide the information. Keep it focused, simple, and objective.

- **Be Clear and Concise:** Avoid overwhelming detail. Use plain language, avoiding technical jargon where possible (or explaining it clearly if necessary). Offer information in small chunks.
- **Be Neutral:** Present the information as objective fact, without persuasive language, warnings, or judgment. Focus on *what is*, not *what they should do*.
    - *Less Neutral:* "You really need to understand that this medication is essential to prevent a heart attack, so you absolutely must take it."
    - *More Neutral:* "This medication helps to relax the blood vessels, which lowers blood pressure and reduces the strain on your heart. Studies show it significantly lowers the risk of heart attack and stroke for many people."
- **Relate to Patient's Goals (Optional but helpful):** If possible, link the information back to concerns or goals the patient has already expressed.
    - *"You mentioned earlier wanting more energy. One thing that can sometimes help with energy levels when managing diabetes is..."*
- **Use Aids Thoughtfully:** Pamphlets, diagrams, or videos can be useful, but introduce them within the

EPE framework. "Would you find it helpful to look at a diagram showing how this works?"

The goal here is straightforward delivery of relevant information, keeping it brief enough for the patient to easily digest.

Step 3: Elicit - Ask for the patients reaction understanding or takeaway

This final "Elicit" step is essential and often overlooked in traditional education. After providing the information, immediately check back with the patient to understand their response. What did they hear? What do they make of it? How does it land with them?

- **Check Understanding/Reaction:** Use open questions.
    - *"What are your thoughts on that?"*
    - *"What does that information mean to you?"*
    - *"How does that fit with your own experience or understanding?"*
    - *"What questions does that raise for you?"*
    - *"Given that information, what makes sense to you as a next step?"*
    - *"Could you tell me in your own words what you heard me say, just so I know I was clear?"* (Use this "teach-back" method carefully, framing it as checking *your* clarity, not testing *their* knowledge).

This step allows you to:

- Assess their comprehension and correct any misunderstandings immediately.
- Hear their emotional reaction to the information.
- Understand how they are integrating the information with their own beliefs and values.
- Transition back into exploring their perspective and potential next steps, guided by the new information.

It closes the loop, ensuring the information exchange was truly a two-way street and provides a natural bridge back to collaborative planning or further exploration.

The EPE Cycle

EPE isn't necessarily a one-time process in a conversation. You might cycle through it multiple times as different topics arise or as the patient asks further questions. Elicit -> Provide -> Elicit -> Explore -> Elicit -> Provide -> Elicit...

Case Study: Nurse Garcia Explains A1c Results using EPE

Nurse Garcia is meeting with Mr. Peters, who has type 2 diabetes. His recent A1c result is higher than desired.

Nurse Garcia: "Mr. Peters, the results from your recent blood work are back, including the A1c test. **Before we look at the number, what's your understanding of what the A1c test tells us?**" (**Elicit** - Knowledge)

Mr. Peters: "It's… something about my average sugar over time, right? Like a few months?"

Nurse Garcia: "Exactly, you've got it. It gives us a picture of your average blood sugar control over the past 2-3 months.

Would you like to talk about your specific result now and what it might mean?" (**Affirmation, Elicit** - Permission)

Mr. Peters: "Yeah, okay. I'm a bit nervous."

Nurse Garcia: "It's understandable to feel nervous. (Empathy). Your A1c result this time is 8.8%. Generally, for many people with diabetes, a goal is often below 7% to reduce the risk of long-term complications like eye or kidney problems." (**Provide** - Clear, neutral information linking result to general goal/risk).

Nurse Garcia: "**What are your thoughts when you hear that number, 8.8%?**" (**Elicit** - Reaction/Understanding)

Mr. Peters: "Well, it's higher than I hoped. I guess I haven't been doing as well as I thought with my diet. Does this mean I need more medication?"

Nurse Garcia: "That's a really good question. (Affirmation). It tells us that blood sugars have been running higher on average, and exploring medication adjustments might be one option to discuss with the doctor. **What else comes to mind for you when thinking about managing your sugars? Are there other things you'd be interested in discussing, like diet or activity strategies?**" (**Provide** - Acknowledging one option, **Elicit** - Interest/Priorities)

Mr. Peters: "Maybe we could talk about diet again. I struggle with lunches at work."

Nurse Garcia: "Okay. So, focusing on strategies for work lunches feels like a helpful place to start for you right now. (Reflection/Summary). **What have you already tried or thought about regarding lunches?**" (**Elicit** - Knowledge/Experience)

Notice how Nurse Garcia uses EPE. She checks Mr. Peters' understanding first, asks permission, provides the result neutrally with context, immediately asks for his reaction, acknowledges his concerns, and then uses his response to guide the next step, eliciting his interest before potentially providing more information about diet strategies. The conversation remains collaborative and focused on Mr. Peters' perspective and priorities.

Nursing Focus Using EPE for Common Tasks

EPE is highly adaptable for many routine nursing tasks involving information exchange:

- **Explaining Conditions:**
    - E: "What have doctors told you about your heart failure before?" / "Would you like me to briefly explain how heart failure affects the body?"
    - P: (Provide clear, simple explanation focused on key mechanisms and symptoms).
    - E: "What does that explanation make you think about?" / "How does that fit with what you've been experiencing?"
- **Discussing Treatment Options:**
    - E: "We have a couple of options for managing this pain. What are your thoughts on using medication versus trying physical therapy first?" / "Would you like me to outline the potential pros and cons of each approach?"

- P: (Provide balanced, neutral information about each option).
- E: "Hearing that, which approach feels like a better fit for you right now, or what other questions do you have?"

- **Explaining Medication Side Effects:**
    - E: "This medication can sometimes cause side effects. What concerns do you have about that?" / "Would it be helpful to talk about the common side effects and how likely they are?"
    - P: (Provide specific information about common side effects and their management, perhaps mentioning less common but serious ones).
    - E: "What are your thoughts about those possible side effects?" / "How concerning does that sound to you?"

- **Teaching Self-Management Techniques (e.g., inhaler use, wound care):**
    - E: "What's your experience been with using inhalers like this one?" / "Would you like me to demonstrate the steps for using it correctly?"
    - P: (Demonstrate the technique clearly).
    - E: "What did you notice as I went through those steps?" / "How about you give it a try now, and we can walk through it together?" (Teach-back).

Using EPE consistently helps ensure patients are active participants in their learning. It increases the likelihood they understand the information, feel their concerns are addressed, and can make informed decisions aligned with their own values and circumstances. It turns education from a monologue into a dialogue.

Sharing Wisely Key Takeaways

- Providing information is a key nursing role, but *how* it's done matters greatly in MI.

- Avoid the "Information Dump," which can lead to overload, anxiety, and resistance.

- The **Elicit-Provide-Elicit (EPE)** method offers a collaborative, MI-consistent way to share information.

- **Step 1: Elicit** - Understand the patient's current knowledge/interest and **ask permission** before providing information.

- **Step 2: Provide** - Offer information **clearly, concisely, and neutrally**, avoiding jargon and persuasion. Keep it brief.

- **Step 3: Elicit** - Immediately ask for the patient's **reaction, understanding, or takeaway** using open questions. Check comprehension.

- EPE respects patient autonomy, tailors information, improves understanding, and maintains collaboration.

- Use EPE cyclically for various nursing tasks like explaining conditions, treatment options, side effects, and self-management techniques.

We've covered the MI mindset, the core OARS skills, how to work with change talk and discord, and how to share information effectively using EPE. Now, the conversation often turns toward action. How do you help patients move from *talking* about change to actually *planning* for it? Chapter 6 focuses on collaborative goal setting and action planning, ensuring the patient remains in the driver's seat as they map out their next steps.

Chapter 6: From Talk to Action- Collaborative Goal Setting and Planning

The conversation has shifted. Through skillful use of MI, you've journeyed with the patient through their ambivalence. You've listened attentively, reflected their perspective, evoked their own reasons for change (change talk), and navigated moments of discord respectfully. Now, you might sense a readiness, a leaning toward action. The patient may be moving from "if" or "why" to "how." This is the crucial transition point from exploring change to planning for it. However, jumping into planning too soon, before the patient is truly ready, can backfire, reigniting ambivalence or creating discord. Conversely, missing the window when a patient *is* ready can lead to lost momentum. This chapter focuses on recognizing readiness, collaboratively developing specific action plans, anticipating roadblocks, and solidifying commitment—all while keeping the patient firmly in the driver's seat.

Knowing When to Plan Recognizing readiness cues

Timing is key. How do you know when it's appropriate to shift the conversation toward making a concrete plan? Look and listen for signals—readiness cues—that suggest the patient is moving from contemplation toward preparation or action. These cues often include:

1. **Decreased Sustain Talk/Discord:** The patient voices fewer arguments for staying the same and fewer signs of interactional friction (arguing, ignoring). The overall tone feels more open and collaborative.

2. **Increased Change Talk:** You hear more mobilizing change talk (Commitment, Activation, Taking Steps - CAT) alongside the preparatory talk (Desire, Ability, Reason, Need - DARN). They might say things like, "I think I'm ready to try something," or "I'm going to have to do X."

3. **Questions About Change:** The patient starts asking practical questions about *how* to make the change. *"So, what kinds of exercises would be safe for me?" "How exactly does that medication patch work?" "Where could I find healthier recipes?"*

4. **Envisioning:** The patient talks about what life might be like *after* the change has been made. *"It would be great to walk up those stairs without getting winded." "Maybe I could save enough money for a vacation if I quit smoking."*

5. **Experimenting/Taking Small Steps:** The patient reports having already tried something related to the change goal, even if minor. *"I actually chose water instead of soda yesterday." "I looked up the gym schedule."*

When you notice these cues accumulating, it's often a good signal that the patient might be ready to talk specifics. A simple way to test the waters is with a **key question** that summarizes the situation and invites consideration of next steps.

- *"We've talked a lot about the pros and cons of [making the change]. What do you think you might do now?"*

- *"Given everything we've discussed, what seems like the most logical next step for you?"*
- *"You sound like you're leaning more toward [making the change]. How might you go about it?"*
- *"Where does this leave you?"*

Listen carefully to the response. If the patient readily engages with planning ideas, proceed. If they hesitate, backtrack, or express significant ambivalence again, don't push. Simply reflect their hesitation ("It sounds like you're still feeling unsure about the 'how'") and return to exploring their perspective. Planning must occur *with* the patient, not *at* them.

Key Questions Moving from general goals to specific plans

Once readiness is established, the planning phase begins. This isn't about you dictating a plan; it's about using evocative open questions to help the patient construct their *own* plan. The goal is to move from vague intentions ("I want to eat healthier") to concrete, actionable steps.

Useful key questions during planning include:

- **Goal Clarification:**
    - *"What specific change are you thinking about making?"*
    - *"If you were successful with this, what would things look like?"*
    - *"What would be a realistic first step for you?"*
- **Exploring Options:**

- o "What are some different ways you could approach this?"
- o "What have you tried before that worked, even partly?"
- o "What ideas do you have about how to start?"

- **Detailing the Plan:**
    - o "Specifically, what will you do?"
    - o "When will you do it?"
    - o "How often?"
    - o "Where will this happen?"
    - o "What support might you need?" (From others, resources, etc.)

- **Assessing Confidence:**
    - o "On a scale of 0 to 10, how confident are you that you can carry out this specific plan?"
    - o (If confidence is low, e.g., below 7) "What makes it a [lower number] rather than a zero?" (Elicits ability/strengths) "What would need to happen for that number to be higher?" (Problem-solves barriers, may lead to adjusting the plan to be more achievable).

Your role is to guide this process, helping the patient think through the details and craft a plan that feels manageable and personally relevant. Use reflections and summaries to keep the plan clear and reinforce their commitment language.

Developing a SMART(er) Plan Specific Measurable Achievable Relevant Time-bound and patient-driven

A common framework for effective goal setting is **SMART**. A good plan is:

- **S**pecific: Clearly defines what needs to be done. Avoid vague goals like "exercise more." Instead, aim for "walk briskly around the block."
- **M**easurable: Defines how you will know the goal is met. How much? How often? How long? "Walk briskly around the block **three times**."
- **A**chievable (or **A**ttainable): The goal should be realistic given the patient's current abilities, resources, and circumstances. Starting small is often best. Is walking around the block feasible, or should it be walking to the end of the driveway first? Confidence scaling helps here.
- **R**elevant (or **R**ealistic): The goal should align with the patient's broader values and health objectives. Does this specific action directly contribute to what matters most to them?
- **T**ime-bound (or **T**imely): Specifies a timeframe for action or completion. "Walk briskly around the block three times **this week, starting Tuesday**."

In MI, we add "…**er**"—emphasizing that the plan must be **patient-driven (E**voked)** and collaboratively agreed upon (**R**ecorded or **R**eviewed). The best plan is one the patient creates and owns.

Case Study: Nurse Kevin Helps Plan Activity Increase

Nurse Kevin is working with Mrs. Gable, a 65-year-old woman with osteoarthritis and hypertension who wants to become more active to manage her weight and stiffness. She has expressed readiness.

Nurse Kevin: "Mrs. Gable, you've mentioned wanting to be more active (Desire) because you believe it would help your stiffness and maybe your weight (Reason), and you feel it's important to stay mobile (Need). You sound ready to think about some specific steps. **What kind of activity feels like a possible starting point for you?**" (**Summary** of change talk, **Key Question** inviting planning)

Mrs. Gable: "Well, I used to like swimming, but getting to the pool is hard now. Maybe walking? But my knee hurts."

Nurse Kevin: "**So walking seems like a possibility, but concern about your knee pain is a major factor.**" (**Reflection**). "**What kind of walking, or how much, do you think might be manageable *despite* the knee pain?**" (**Open Question** exploring Achievability)

Mrs. Gable: "I don't know... maybe just down to the corner and back? It's not very far."

Nurse Kevin: "**Okay, so a specific first step could be walking to the corner and back.**" (**Reflection** - Specific). "**How many times a week do you think you could realistically manage that, starting out?**" (**Open Question** - Measurable/Time-bound)

Mrs. Gable: "Hmm. Maybe... three times? Like Monday, Wednesday, Friday?"

Nurse Kevin: "**Walk to the corner and back, three times a week, perhaps Monday, Wednesday, and Friday.**" (**Reflection** - Specific, Measurable, Time-bound). "**Does that feel like something you could achieve this coming week?**" (**Open Question** - checking Achievability)

Mrs. Gable: "Yes, I think I could do that. It's not too much."

Nurse Kevin: "**And how does this specific step—walking to the corner and back three times this week—fit with your overall goal of managing stiffness and weight?**" (**Open Question** - checking Relevance)

Mrs. Gable: "Well, it's a start! Better than just sitting."

Nurse Kevin: "**Okay. So the plan is: Walk to the corner and back on Monday, Wednesday, and Friday this week.**" (**Summary** - confirming SMART plan). "**On a scale of 0 to 10, where 10 is completely confident, how confident are you that you can carry out this plan this week?**" (**Open Question** - assessing Confidence)

Mrs. Gable: "Oh, probably an 8 or 9. It feels doable."

Nurse Kevin: "**An 8 or 9, that's great! What gives you that level of confidence?**" (**Open Question** - eliciting strengths/Ability)

Mrs. Gable: "Because it's short, and I can pick the time of day when my knee feels best."

Nurse Kevin has guided Mrs. Gable to create a SMART plan that feels owned and achievable, setting her up for potential success.

Troubleshooting and Anticipating Barriers Even the best plans hit snags

Things rarely go exactly as planned. Part of effective planning is anticipating potential obstacles and brainstorming solutions *in advance*. This builds realism and self-efficacy—the patient sees that challenges are expected and can be managed.

- **Ask About Barriers:**
    - *"What might get in the way of carrying out this plan?"*
    - *"What challenges have come up when you've tried similar things before?"*
    - *"Thinking about the week ahead, what could make it difficult to stick with this?"*
- **Brainstorm Solutions Collaboratively:** Once potential barriers are identified, use open questions to elicit the patient's ideas for overcoming them.
    - *"If [the barrier] happens, how might you handle it?"*
    - *"What strategies could you use to deal with [the challenge]?"*
    - *"Who or what could support you if things get tough?"*
    - *"What would be a backup plan if the original plan isn't possible on a particular day?"*

Continuing Case Study: Mrs. Gable's Barriers

Nurse Kevin: **"We have this plan for the walking. Sometimes life throws us curveballs. What might** possibly get in the way of you doing your walks this week?" (**Open Question** - anticipating barriers)

Mrs. Gable: "Well... bad weather, I suppose. If it's pouring rain, I won't go. Or if my knee is having a really bad day."

Nurse Kevin: "**Okay, so heavy rain or a particularly bad knee day could be obstacles.**" (**Reflection**). "**What could be a Plan B for those days? What might you do instead to stay on track with being active?**" (**Open Question** - brainstorming solutions)

Mrs. Gable: "Hmm. I have some stretching exercises the physical therapist gave me. Maybe I could do those inside instead on those days?"

Nurse Kevin: "**So, if walking isn't possible due to rain or severe pain, your backup plan could be to do your stretching exercises indoors.** That sounds like a flexible approach." (**Summary** of solution, **Affirmation**). "**How confident are you in using that backup plan if needed?**" (**Open Question** - checking confidence in solution)

Mrs. Gable: "Pretty confident. I know how to do the stretches."

By anticipating barriers and co-creating backup plans, the overall plan becomes more robust and Mrs. Gable feels more prepared to handle challenges.

Confirming the Plan and Follow up Solidifying commitment and next steps

Before ending the conversation, it's important to clearly summarize the final plan and confirm the patient's commitment. This reinforces the decision and clarifies expectations for follow-up.

- **Summarize the Final Plan:** Briefly restate the specific actions, timing, frequency, and any backup plans agreed upon.
    - *"Okay, so just to recap, the plan is to walk to the corner and back on Monday, Wednesday, and Friday this week. If weather or knee pain prevents the walk, you'll do your indoor stretching exercises instead. Does that sound right?"*
- **Confirm Commitment:** You might use a final mobilizing change talk question.
    - *"So, is this something you intend to do?"*
    - *"How ready are you to put this plan into action?"*
- **Arrange Follow-up:** Discuss how progress will be monitored or discussed.
    - *"How would you like to check in about how this plan is going? Would you prefer a call next week, or should we discuss it at your next scheduled visit?"*
    - *"Perhaps you could jot down how the walks go, and we can look at it together next time?"*

This confirmation step provides closure to the planning process and sets the stage for accountability and ongoing support.

Nursing Focus Helping patients create realistic action steps

Your role in planning isn't to prescribe the perfect plan, but to facilitate the patient's process of creating a plan that is **meaningful, realistic, and achievable** *for them*. This applies across various nursing contexts:

- **Managing Chronic Illness:** Helping a patient with diabetes plan *how* they will incorporate regular blood sugar monitoring into their day, or *how* a patient with COPD will use their inhalers correctly and consistently. The plan needs to fit *their* routine and address *their* perceived barriers.

- **Adopting Healthier Habits:** Guiding someone wanting to improve their diet to identify *one specific change* they feel confident making (e.g., swapping sugary drinks for water at lunch), rather than attempting a complete overhaul. Helping someone plan *how* they will manage cravings when quitting smoking.

- **Adhering to Treatment:** Collaborating with a patient struggling with medication adherence to brainstorm *specific strategies* for remembering (pill organizers, alarms, linking to daily routines) and creating a plan *they choose* to try. Addressing concerns about side effects and planning *how* they will manage them or communicate with the provider.

The key is always **collaboration** and **patient autonomy**. A plan developed *by* the patient, even if it seems small to you, is far more likely to be implemented than a "perfect" plan imposed *on* them. Start small, build confidence, celebrate small successes, and adjust the plan as needed over time.

Action Planning Essentials

- Transition to planning when you observe **readiness cues** (less sustain talk, more change talk, questions about change, envisioning, taking steps).

- Use **key open questions** to move from general goals to specific actions, clarifying the what, when, where, and how.

- Guide the patient to develop a **SMART(er)** plan: Specific, Measurable, Achievable, Relevant, Time-bound, and crucially, **patient-driven (Evoked & Reviewed)**.

- Actively **anticipate barriers** and collaboratively brainstorm solutions or backup plans.

- Assess **patient confidence** in the plan using scaling questions; adjust the plan if confidence is low.

- **Confirm the final plan** clearly and discuss follow-up arrangements.

- In all nursing contexts, focus on helping patients create **realistic, achievable first steps** that they own, rather than prescribing complex regimens.

We've now covered the core spirit, skills, and processes of MI, from initial engagement through collaborative planning. But how does this all look woven into the fabric of your actual workday? Chapter 7 brings MI to life by demonstrating its application in brief, common nursing scenarios you likely encounter regularly, showing how these techniques can be integrated efficiently and effectively.

Chapter 7: CMI in Motion- Applying Techniques in Common Nursing Scenarios

Theory is one thing; practice is another. We've discussed the spirit of Motivational Interviewing, sharpened our OARS skills, learned to listen for change talk, navigated discord, exchanged information effectively, and collaborated on planning. Now, let's put it all together. How does MI actually *look and sound* during the fast-paced, varied encounters that make up a nurse's day? This chapter focuses on applying MI principles and techniques within typical nursing workflows, demonstrating how even brief interventions can be impactful. We'll examine several common scenarios, providing sample dialogue snippets and highlighting the MI strategies being used. The goal isn't to provide rigid scripts, but to illustrate the fluid application of MI in real-world nursing contexts.

Brief MI Interventions 5-15 minutes

A frequent concern nurses raise is time. "MI sounds great, but I don't have 30 minutes for counseling." The good news is, you don't need it. While longer MI sessions exist, the core principles and skills can be effectively integrated into interactions lasting just **5 to 15 minutes**. This is often called **Brief MI** or **MI-informed care**. It's not about doing *more*, but about doing what you already do *differently*. It involves:

- **Adopting the MI Spirit:** Approaching the interaction with Partnership, Acceptance, Compassion, and Evocation.

- **Using OARS Selectively:** Employing Open questions, Affirmations, Reflections, and Summaries strategically, even just a few times.
- **Listening for Change Talk:** Tuning your ears to hear the patient's own motivation.
- **Rolling with Discord:** Responding non-confrontationally if friction arises.
- **Using EPE for Information:** Sharing advice or education collaboratively when needed.
- **Focusing on a Specific Target:** Often, a brief intervention will focus on one particular behavior or aspect of ambivalence.

Think of it as weaving MI threads into the existing fabric of your nursing care—during assessments, medication reviews, patient education, discharge planning, or even brief check-ins.

Let's look at some scenarios. (Note: Dialogue snippets are illustrative, not exhaustive).

Scenario 1 Medication Adherence Primary Care Chronic Disease

Situation: Nurse practitioner Alex is seeing Mr. Thompson, a 68-year-old man with hypertension and high cholesterol, for a follow-up. His blood pressure is still elevated despite prescriptions for Lisinopril and Atorvastatin.

Alex (NP): "Mr. Thompson, good to see you. Your blood pressure reading today is 158/94, which is still higher than our goal. **How have things been going with taking the**

Lisinopril and Atorvastatin each day since your last visit?" (**Open Question**)

Mr. Thompson: "Oh, you know... mostly okay. I try to remember." (Vague, hints at non-adherence).

Alex: "**So, taking them consistently every single day has been a bit challenging.**" (**Reflection**)

Mr. Thompson: "Yeah. Sometimes I just forget the evening one—the cholesterol pill. Mornings are easier with my breakfast."

Alex: "**You've found a good system for remembering the morning Lisinopril by linking it to breakfast.**" (**Affirmation** of existing strategy). "**But the evening Atorvastatin gets missed sometimes.**" (**Reflection**). "**What makes the evening dose harder to remember?**" (**Open Question** exploring barrier).

Mr. Thompson: "I don't know... I eat dinner at different times, sometimes I fall asleep in the recliner... there's no set routine like breakfast."

Alex: "**So the lack of a consistent evening routine makes it easy for the Atorvastatin to slip through the cracks.**" (**Reflection**). "**It takes real effort to add a new medication into a varied schedule.**" (**Affirmation**). "**We know keeping cholesterol down is important for preventing heart attack and stroke.** (Brief Provide - linking to benefit). **What ideas do you have, or what have you considered, that might help you remember that evening dose more reliably?**" (**Open Question** - eliciting solutions).

Mr. Thompson: "Maybe... I could set an alarm on my phone? Around 8 pm?"

Alex: "**Setting an 8 pm phone alarm is one possibility.**" (**Reflection**). "**How likely would you be to follow through with that idea? What might get in the way?**" (**Open Question** - exploring commitment/barriers).

Mr. Thompson: "I'd probably do it if the alarm went off. Unless I left my phone in the other room."

Alex: "**So the alarm seems like a good prompt, as long as your phone is nearby.**" (**Reflection**). "**What could ensure your phone is usually nearby around 8 pm?**" (**Open Question** - problem-solving).

Mr. Thompson: "I could make a point to put it on the end table beside my recliner after dinner."

Alex: "**Okay, so the plan taking shape is: Set a daily 8 pm alarm on your phone specifically for the Atorvastatin, and make a habit of putting the phone on the end table after dinner.**" (**Summary** of plan). "**How does that plan sound to you as something to try for the next month?**" (**Open Question** - checking buy-in).

Mr. Thompson: "Yeah, I can try that. It's worth a shot." (**Activation/Commitment**).

Alex: "**Great. You're willing to give that strategy a try.** (**Reflection**). Let's check back at your next appointment and see how it worked out." (**Affirmation, Confirming follow-up**).

MI Elements Used: Open questions to explore adherence and barriers, Reflections to show understanding, Affirmations for existing strategies and willingness, collaborative Problem-Solving, Summarizing the patient's plan, Checking for commitment. The focus was narrow (evening medication) and the exchange likely took only 5-7 minutes within the larger appointment.

Scenario 2 Discussing Lifestyle Changes Diet Exercise Smoking Community Health Primary Care

Situation: Nurse Maya, a community health nurse, is doing a home visit with Brenda, a 45-year-old single mother who smokes and wants to lose weight but feels overwhelmed.

Maya: "Brenda, thanks for having me over. We've talked before about your interest in losing some weight and maybe cutting back on smoking. **Where are those things sitting for you today?**" (**Open Question**, checking current status/priorities).

Brenda: "Oh gosh. Still want to. Still doing neither! (Laughs). I feel stuck. Work is crazy, the kids need me... I grab fast food a lot. And smoking... it's my stress relief."

Maya: "**It sounds like you're juggling a ton, and even though you want to make changes for your health, finding the time, energy, and alternative coping strategies feels overwhelming right now.**" (**Complex Reflection** capturing feeling/dilemma).

Brenda: "Exactly! Like, where do I even start?"

Maya: "**That's a great question – 'Where to start?' It shows you're thinking about possibilities, even with all the challenges.**" (**Affirmation** reframing the question positively). "**Of all the things related to health – eating habits, activity, smoking – what feels like it might be the *most* important area for you to focus on, or perhaps the *easiest* one to tackle first?**" (**Open Question** - helping prioritize).

Brenda: "Hmm. Maybe the smoking? I hate the smell on my clothes, and it costs so much. But quitting seems impossible."

Maya: "**So, reducing or quitting smoking feels important because of the smell and the cost, but the idea of actually doing it feels incredibly daunting, maybe impossible from where you sit today.**" (**Double-Sided Reflection** capturing ambivalence).

Brenda: "Yeah."

Maya: "**What makes it feel impossible right now?**" (**Open Question** - exploring barriers/sustain talk).

Brenda: "It's my main way to cope with stress. If I didn't smoke when I got stressed, I don't know what I'd do."

Maya: "**So finding other ways to manage stress is a key piece of the puzzle if you were to cut back or quit smoking.**" (**Reflection** identifying a key need). "**Have you ever thought about or tried other stress-relief techniques?**" (**Open Question** exploring alternatives/past experience).

Brenda: "Someone told me about deep breathing, but it sounds silly."

Maya: "**You're skeptical about deep breathing.** (Reflection). **Some people find it helpful, others don't. Would you be willing to just try one quick, simple breathing exercise with me right now, just to see what it's like? It takes about 30 seconds.**" (**Normalizing, Elicit** - permission for experiment/Activation).

Brenda: (Hesitantly) "Okay, I guess. What do I have to lose?"

(Maya briefly guides Brenda through a simple diaphragmatic breath).

Maya: "**What did you notice during those few breaths?**" (**Open Question** - eliciting reaction).

Brenda: "It was... calmer than I expected. Didn't solve anything, but... calmer."

Maya: "**So it felt a bit calming, even if it wasn't a magic wand.**" (**Reflection**). "**How might incorporating something simple like that, maybe just for a minute when stress hits, fit in as one possible tool alongside smoking, or maybe even instead of reaching for a cigarette sometimes?**" (**Open Question** exploring possibility/linking to goal).

MI Elements Used: Open questions to check priorities and explore barriers/solutions, Reflections (complex, double-sided) to explore ambivalence and show empathy, Affirmations to build confidence, using EPE implicitly to suggest trying an exercise, focusing on one small potential step (trying breathing) rather than demanding quitting. This conversation respects Brenda's feeling of being overwhelmed while gently exploring one potential coping alternative.

Scenario 3 Engaging a Patient with Low Motivation Mental Health General

Situation: Nurse Chen works on an inpatient mental health unit. Liam, a 28-year-old man experiencing depression, rarely attends group therapy sessions despite encouragement.

Chen: "Liam, I notice you haven't been making it to the group therapy sessions recently. **What's been going on for you** around group time?" (**Behavioral observation, Open Question** exploring perspective).

Liam: (Shrugs) "Don't feel like it. It's pointless."

Chen: "**From your perspective right now, going to group feels pointless, like it wouldn't help.**" (**Reflection**).

Liam: "Yeah. Just people talking about their stupid problems."

Chen: "**So you don't see the value in hearing others talk about their issues.**" (**Reflection**). "**What, if anything, *do* you hope to get out of being here in the hospital?**" (**Open Question** - shifting focus to broader goals/values).

Liam: "Get out of here. Feel less... heavy."

Chen: "**Feeling less heavy and eventually leaving the hospital are your main goals right now.**" (**Reflection**). "**What do you think needs to happen for you to start feeling less heavy?**" (**Open Question** linking goal to potential actions).

Liam: (Shrugs again) "I don't know. Sleep forever?"

Chen: "**It sounds like you're feeling really hopeless, maybe even thinking things won't get better.**" (**Complex Reflection** - capturing deep feeling). "**That must be an incredibly difficult place to be.**" (**Empathy**).

Liam: (Quietly) "It sucks."

Chen: "**It really sucks.**" (**Simple Reflection**). "**Liam, you've been through tough times before and found ways to cope. You're incredibly resilient just by being here and talking now.**" (**Affirmation** highlighting strength/coping). "**I know group doesn't feel right for you now. Is there *anything* else, even something small, that sometimes helps lift that heavy feeling, even just a tiny bit? Music? Walking outside? Talking one-on-one?" (**Acknowledging resistance**, **Open Question** exploring alternative positive actions/past successes).

Liam: "Sometimes music helps. A little."

Chen: "**Music helps a bit sometimes.**" (**Reflection**). "**Would you be open to making sure you have access to your music player and headphones today, maybe aiming to listen for at least 15-20 minutes?**" (**Elicit** permission/Activation for a small, patient-identified step).

MI Elements Used: Starting with empathy and reflection of the patient's negative perspective ("pointless"), avoiding arguing about group benefits (rolling with discord), shifting focus to the patient's broader goals ("get out," "feel less heavy"), deep reflection of hopelessness, affirming resilience, exploring alternative small steps the patient identifies (music), seeking collaboration on one achievable action. The immediate goal isn't group attendance, but engaging Liam in *any* positive action he feels willing to try.

Scenario 4 Supporting Self-Management in Chronic Illness Diabetes COPD Heart Failure

Situation: Nurse practitioner Simone is reviewing self-management with Mrs. Diaz, a 72-year-old woman with COPD who sometimes forgets to use her inhalers as prescribed.

Simone (NP): "Mrs. Diaz, we know using your inhalers regularly is key to managing your COPD symptoms. **Tell me a bit about how you incorporate them into your daily routine.**" (**Open Question** exploring current behavior).

Mrs. Diaz: "Oh, the blue one (rescue inhaler) I use when I get breathless. The purple one (controller inhaler)... I try to remember it morning and night, but sometimes I forget, especially the evening one."

Simone: "**So you're very clear on using the blue rescue inhaler when needed.** (Affirmation). **And you intend to use the purple controller inhaler twice daily, but consistency, especially in the evening, can be tricky.**" (**Reflection** highlighting intention and challenge).

Mrs. Diaz: "Yes. Sometimes I just feel okay, so I think maybe I don't need it."

Simone: "**There are times you feel pretty good and question if the purple inhaler is necessary at that moment.**" (**Reflection**). "**What do you understand about how the purple controller inhaler works differently from the blue rescue one?**" (**Elicit** - knowledge using EPE).

Mrs. Diaz: "The blue one is for immediate help. The purple one is... long-term? To prevent things?"

Simone: "**That's a great way to put it.** (Affirmation). The blue one opens your airways quickly when you feel breathless. The purple one works over time to reduce inflammation in your airways, making those breathless episodes less likely to happen in the first place. It works best when used consistently every day, even when you feel well, to keep that inflammation down." (**Provide** - clear, neutral info). "**What are your thoughts on hearing that explanation?**" (**Elicit** - reaction/understanding).

Mrs. Diaz: "Okay, that makes sense. So it's like prevention. I guess I should try harder to remember it." (**Reason**, potential **Commitment**).

Simone: "**It sounds like understanding the preventative role makes taking it consistently feel more important to you.**" (**Reflection** linking understanding to need/commitment). "**You mentioned the evening dose is sometimes forgotten. What might make it easier to remember that specific dose?**" (**Open Question** inviting solutions).

Mrs. Diaz: "Maybe if I kept it right on my nightstand? I always see my pills there before bed."

Simone: "**Keeping the purple inhaler with your other nighttime medications on the nightstand could be a good visual reminder.**" (**Reflection**). "**How confident are you that making that one change—moving the inhaler—would help you remember the evening dose most days?**" (**Open Question** assessing confidence in strategy).

Mrs. Diaz: "Oh, quite confident! If it's right there, I'll see it."

Simone: "**Excellent. So the plan is to move the purple inhaler to your nightstand tonight to help remember that evening dose.** (Summary). Let's see how that works over the next few weeks." (**Confirming plan and follow-up**).

MI Elements Used: Open questions to explore routine and solutions, Reflections to ensure understanding, Affirmations for correct understanding and effort, EPE framework to explain medication function clearly and check understanding, focusing on a specific patient-generated solution (moving the inhaler), assessing confidence.

These scenarios illustrate that MI isn't a rigid protocol but a flexible, adaptable communication style. By weaving in the spirit and selected OARS skills, even brief interactions can become more collaborative, patient-centered, and effective in supporting health behavior change.

Applying MI Key Points

- Motivational Interviewing can be effectively used in **brief interventions** (5-15 minutes) within routine nursing care.[4]
- Brief MI involves applying the **MI spirit**, using **OARS selectively**, listening for **change talk**, **rolling with discord**, and using **EPE** for information sharing.
- **Scenario 1 (Medication Adherence):** Focused on exploring barriers to one specific medication dose and collaboratively finding a patient-generated solution (phone alarm).
- **Scenario 2 (Lifestyle Changes):** Navigated overwhelm by helping the patient prioritize, exploring ambivalence about smoking using reflections, and inviting experimentation with one small alternative coping strategy (breathing exercise).
- **Scenario 3 (Low Motivation):** Used empathy and reflection to engage a withdrawn patient, avoided arguing, shifted focus to patient goals, affirmed strengths, and collaborated on one small, patient-chosen positive action (listening to music).
- **Scenario 4 (Chronic Illness Self-Management):** Used EPE to clarify medication purpose, linked understanding to importance, explored barriers to adherence, and supported a specific, patient-designed reminder strategy (moving inhaler).

- The key is fluidly applying MI principles and skills to make interactions more collaborative and patient-centered, even when time is limited.

Seeing MI in action across these scenarios highlights its adaptability. But the reality of nursing often involves significant time pressures and workflow demands. How can you consistently weave these techniques into your practice when the clock is always ticking? Chapter 8 offers practical tips and strategies specifically for integrating MI into time-constrained nursing environments.

Chapter 8: Adding MI into Your Workflow-Tips for Time-Constrained Encounters

The scenarios in the previous chapter demonstrated MI in action, but often in somewhat contained moments. The reality of nursing, as you know all too well, is frequently fragmented, fast-paced, and demanding. Bells ring, emergencies arise, documentation calls, and patients have immediate needs. The persistent question remains: "How can I possibly fit this MI approach into *my* chaotic workday?" It's a fair question, grounded in the genuine pressures of clinical practice. This chapter addresses that concern directly, offering practical strategies to make MI feasible—not as an add-on burden, but as an integrated, efficient way to communicate—even when minutes are scarce.

MI Isnt About More Time Its About Better Time

Let's reframe the time issue. While learning any new skill takes initial effort, the goal of integrating MI isn't necessarily to spend *more* time with each patient. It's about making the time you *do* spend more **effective and productive**. Consider the time currently spent:

- Re-explaining instructions patients didn't grasp initially.
- Addressing complications from non-adherence.
- Dealing with patient frustration or complaints stemming from feeling unheard.

- Repeating the same persuasive arguments that haven't worked before.
- Managing the emotional toll of feeling ineffective or disconnected.

MI, used skillfully, can actually *reduce* some of this wasted time and effort in the long run. How?

- **By reducing discord:** Rolling with resistance avoids lengthy arguments or standoffs.
- **By increasing clarity:** Using reflections and EPE ensures mutual understanding, reducing the need for repeated explanations.
- **By enhancing engagement:** When patients feel heard and partnered with, they are more likely to participate actively in their care and problem-solving.
- **By fostering intrinsic motivation:** Tapping into the patient's *own* reasons for change leads to more sustainable effort than relying solely on external prompts from you.
- **By improving rapport:** Stronger relationships make all interactions smoother and more efficient.

So, the investment is in shifting the *quality* of your communication minutes, aiming for interactions that are less about pushing and more about partnering. This often yields better results with potentially less struggle – a more efficient use of your valuable time.

Identifying High-Yield Moments for MI Assessments key education points moments of patient reflection

You don't need to use MI constantly with every patient. The key is to be strategic, recognizing moments within your existing workflow where a brief MI intervention can have the most impact. Think of these as **"MI Opportunities"**:

1. **Initial Assessments/Intake:** When gathering patient history or understanding their reason for seeking care, use open questions ("What brings you in today?" "Tell me about...") and reflections to build rapport and understand their perspective from the outset. This sets a collaborative tone.

2. **Key Education Points:** When explaining a new diagnosis, medication, or self-care procedure, use the Elicit-Provide-Elicit (EPE) framework instead of just delivering information. This ensures relevance and understanding.

3. **Discussing Adherence/Behavior:** When checking on medication use, diet, activity, or other health behaviors, use open questions and reflections to explore their experience non-judgmentally ("How has it been going with...?"). Listen for change talk and sustain talk.

4. **Moments of Patient Reflection or Emotion:** When a patient expresses worry, frustration, hope, or ambivalence ("I'm so tired of this," "I really want to get better"), respond with reflective listening. This deepens connection and can open doors to exploring motivation.

5. **Addressing Discrepancies:** When lab results, vital signs, or patient reports don't align with goals (e.g., high A1c, elevated BP, continued smoking despite

desire to quit), use reflections and open questions to explore the discrepancy collaboratively, rather than starting with correction. ("Your A1c is higher than we hoped. What are your thoughts about that?")

6. **Goal Setting/Action Planning:** During discharge planning, care plan updates, or discussions about next steps, use MI principles to ensure goals are patient-driven and realistic (SMARTer goals).

7. **Handling Resistance/Discord:** Any time you feel tension or pushback, see it as a cue to shift into MI mode—reflect, affirm autonomy, roll with it.

By identifying these recurring points in your workflow, you can consciously choose to apply specific MI skills, making the approach feel less like a separate task and more like an enhancement of what you already do.

Using MI Fly Bys Quick applications of OARS or EPE

You don't need to conduct a full MI session in every opportune moment. Often, a quick, targeted application—an "MI Fly-By"—is enough to make a difference. This might involve:

- **A Single Open Question:** Instead of asking "Are you taking your meds?" ask "How's it been going with your medication schedule this week?"

- **A Well-Placed Reflection:** Hearing a patient sigh and say "This is all so overwhelming," respond with "It feels like a lot to handle right now." This simple reflection validates their feeling in seconds.

- **A Quick Affirmation:** Noticing a patient brought their blood sugar log, say "I appreciate you bringing this log in; it really helps us see the trends together."

- **A Mini-EPE:**
    - *Patient:* "What's this new pill for?"
    - *Nurse (Elicit):* "That's the Metoprolol. What have you heard about it, or what questions do you have?"
    - *Patient:* "Isn't it for blood pressure?"
    - *Nurse (Provide):* "Yes, exactly. It helps lower blood pressure and can also help the heart work more easily."
    - *Nurse (Elicit):* "What are your thoughts on adding that in?"

- **A Brief Summary:** At the end of giving instructions, "Okay, so just to quickly recap, you'll call Dr. Smith's office tomorrow to schedule, and continue checking your blood pressure twice daily. Did I get that right?"

These fly-bys might take only 30-60 seconds longer than a purely directive statement or closed question, but they infuse the interaction with the MI spirit, fostering collaboration and understanding without significantly disrupting your flow. String several of these together throughout an encounter, and you're practicing effective brief MI.

Case Study: Nurse Jamal's Efficient MI Fly-Bys

Jamal works on a busy medical-surgical floor. Mrs. Chen is recovering from pneumonia and is anxious about discharge. Jamal needs to review her new inhaler technique.

- *(Jamal enters room, washes hands)* "Good morning, Mrs. Chen. How are you feeling today?" (Standard opening)

- *Mrs. Chen:* "A bit better, but nervous about going home. What if I get sick again?"

- *Jamal:* "**It sounds like you're worried about managing on your own after discharge.**" (**MI Fly-By: Reflection** acknowledging emotion - 10 seconds). "That's understandable. We'll make sure you have a good plan." (Reassurance). "Right now, I need to check your vital signs and listen to your lungs, okay?" (Standard care).

- *(During vital signs) Jamal:* "**What specifically worries you most about going home?**" (**MI Fly-By: Open Question** during routine task - 30 seconds).

- *Mrs. Chen:* "Using that new inhaler correctly. It looks complicated."

- *Jamal:* "**You're concerned about getting the hang of the new inhaler.**" (**MI Fly-By: Reflection** - 5 seconds). "We can definitely practice that. **After I finish listening to your lungs, would you like me to show you the steps again and we can practice together?**" (**MI Fly-By: Elicit** permission using EPE structure - 15 seconds).

- *Mrs. Chen:* "Yes, please."

- *(Later, after assessment) Jamal:* "Okay, let's look at that inhaler. **What do you remember about using it from yesterday's teaching?**" (**MI Fly-By: Elicit** knowledge - 10 seconds).

- *Mrs. Chen:* (Describes some steps correctly, misses one).

- *Jamal:* "**You remembered [correct steps] perfectly!**" (**MI Fly-By: Affirmation** - 5 seconds). "Let me quickly show you that one part about breathing out fully first again." (**Provide**). *(Demonstrates).* "**What do you think about trying it now?**" (**Elicit** reaction/invite practice - 10 seconds).

- *(Mrs. Chen practices).*

- *Jamal:* "**You did that exactly right.**" (**MI Fly-By: Affirmation** - 5 seconds). "**How confident do you feel about using it on your own now?**" (**MI Fly-By: Open Question** checking confidence - 10 seconds).

In this example, Jamal seamlessly integrates quick MI techniques (reflections, open questions, affirmations, EPE elements) into his standard workflow. Each "fly-by" is brief, but together they create a supportive, collaborative interaction focused on Mrs. Chen's specific concerns, likely taking only an extra minute or two overall compared to purely directive teaching.

Focusing on One Small Step Dont try to boil the ocean

When time is limited, resist the urge to address *everything* at once. Patients facing multiple health issues or needing several behavior changes can easily feel overwhelmed. Trying to tackle smoking, diet, exercise, and medication adherence all in one brief encounter is usually counterproductive.

Instead, **collaboratively identify ONE specific, achievable next step** the patient feels most ready or willing to work on.

- **Use Prioritizing Questions:** "Of all the things we've talked about (diet, medication, activity), which one feels like the most important or maybe the easiest one to focus on *right now*?"
- **Listen for Readiness:** Tune into which topic generates the most change talk or patient interest.
- **Aim for Small Wins:** Help the patient define a very small, concrete action they feel confident they can achieve before the next contact. Success with a small step builds self-efficacy for larger changes later. (e.g., "Walk for 5 minutes," "Take medication correctly for 3 days in a row," "Drink one less soda per day").

Focusing the MI effort on collaboratively developing one small, achievable plan is a much more effective use of limited time than superficially touching on multiple complex issues.

Team Collaboration How MI can improve handoffs and team communication about patient goals

MI isn't just for nurse-patient interactions; its principles can enhance team communication too. When the entire team understands and uses MI principles, care becomes more consistent and patient-centered.

- **MI-Informed Handoffs:** Instead of just reporting problems ("Patient non-compliant with meds"), frame the handoff using MI concepts:

- "Mr. Jones expresses **ambivalence** about his new blood pressure medication due to concerns about side effects (dizziness). He voiced **willingness** (Activation) to try taking it at night instead of the morning. **The plan we discussed** is for him to try taking it tonight and report any dizziness tomorrow. His **main goal** is avoiding another hospital stay."
    - This provides richer context about the patient's perspective, motivation, and the collaboratively developed plan.

- **Shared Understanding of Patient Goals:** When care plans incorporate patient-stated goals and motivations (evoked using MI), the entire team can work toward supporting those specific aims, rather than imposing external agendas.

- **Consistent Messaging:** If all team members approach behavior change conversations with MI spirit (partnership, acceptance, compassion, evocation), patients receive consistent, supportive messages, reducing confusion and potential discord.

- **Collaborative Problem-Solving:** Team meetings can use MI principles to discuss challenging cases, focusing on understanding the patient's perspective and brainstorming collaborative strategies, rather than simply labeling patients as "difficult."

Encouraging MI training and practice across the healthcare team can create a more supportive environment for both patients and staff.

Nursing Focus Practical strategies to make MI feasible even on the busiest shifts

Let's distill this into concrete strategies for the time-crunched nurse:

1. **Prepare Your Mindset:** Before starting your shift or entering a patient room, take a moment to intentionally adopt the MI spirit (PACE). Remind yourself: Partner, Accept, Compassion, Evoke.

2. **Identify 1-2 "MI Opportunities" Per Encounter:** Don't try to do it all. Pick one or two high-yield moments (e.g., asking an open question during assessment, using EPE for one key instruction) to consciously apply an MI skill.

3. **Master the "MI Fly-By":** Practice quick, targeted uses of OARS and EPE. Get comfortable with brief reflections that validate emotion, quick affirmations, and asking permission before advising.

4. **Focus on ONE Small Step:** In conversations about change, guide the patient toward identifying and planning one specific, achievable action.

5. **Listen More, Talk Less:** Often, simply listening reflectively takes less time than lengthy persuasion or correction, and is more effective.

6. **Use Wait Time Wisely:** Can you ask an evocative open question while waiting for equipment, during transport, or while performing a routine task?

7. **Embrace Imperfection:** You won't apply MI perfectly every time, especially when busy. Aim for "good enough" integration rather than letting perfectionism

paralyze you. Any step toward more collaborative communication is progress.

8. **Leverage Team Communication:** Use MI language in handoffs to share insights about patient motivation and collaborative plans. Advocate for team-based MI approaches.

9. **Reflect Briefly:** After a challenging interaction, take 30 seconds to ask yourself: "What went well? What could I try differently next time using an MI approach?" This builds skill over time.

Integrating MI into a busy workflow is a skill that develops with practice. Start small, be intentional, focus on high-yield moments, and trust that improving the *quality* of your communication can ultimately lead to more effective and potentially less time-consuming interactions overall.

Making It Work Key Points

- MI aims for **better quality time**, not necessarily more time, potentially saving time by reducing discord and improving adherence long-term.

- Identify **high-yield moments** in your workflow (assessments, education, patient reflection, discrepancies, planning, discord) for brief MI applications.

- Use **"MI Fly-Bys"**: Quick, targeted uses of OARS or EPE (e.g., one reflection, one open question, mini-EPE) integrated into routine tasks.

- When discussing change, focus collaboratively on **one small, specific, achievable step** the patient feels ready for.

- MI principles can enhance **team collaboration** through MI-informed handoffs, shared understanding of patient goals, and consistent messaging.

- Practical strategies include: adopting the MI mindset, identifying key opportunities, mastering fly-bys, focusing on one step, listening more, using wait time, embracing imperfection, leveraging team communication, and brief self-reflection.

- Consistent, intentional practice makes MI feasible even on the busiest shifts.

Making MI work within your workflow is one challenge; sustaining the practice and yourself is another. Engaging deeply with patients about behavior change can be emotionally demanding. Chapter 9 addresses the crucial topic of self-care and preventing burnout, exploring how MI principles and reflective practice can help you maintain your effectiveness and well-being over the long haul.

Chapter 9: Sustaining Your Practice- Self-Reflection and Preventing Burnout

You've come this far. You understand the spirit and principles of Motivational Interviewing, you're practicing the OARS skills, navigating challenging conversations, and finding ways to weave MI into your demanding workflow. This is significant progress. But using MI effectively isn't just about mastering techniques; it's also about sustaining *yourself* in this work. Supporting patients through the often slow and non-linear process of behavior change requires patience, empathy, and resilience. It involves managing complex emotions—both the patient's and your own. Without conscious attention to your own well-being and professional growth, the very empathy that makes MI effective can lead to burnout. This chapter focuses on strategies for maintaining your enthusiasm, effectiveness, and personal balance while using MI long-term.

The Emotional Labor of Behavior Change Support

Nursing, by its nature, involves significant emotional labor—the process of managing your feelings and expressions to fulfill the emotional requirements of the job. When you engage with patients using MI, this emotional labor intensifies. You are:

- **Deeply Listening:** Trying to understand the world from another's perspective, including their struggles, fears, and hopes.

- **Managing Your Reactions:** Intentionally avoiding the "righting reflex," judgment, or frustration, even when faced with difficult behaviors or discord.

- **Holding Hope:** Maintaining belief in the patient's capacity for change, sometimes even when they struggle to believe in themselves.

- **Containing Difficult Emotions:** Sitting with patients' sadness, anger, fear, or despair without becoming overwhelmed yourself.

- **Navigating Ambivalence:** Tolerating the patient's uncertainty and the non-linear path of change without pushing for premature resolution.

This requires significant emotional regulation and psychological energy. While incredibly rewarding when successful, it can also be draining, especially when progress is slow or setbacks occur. Recognizing this inherent emotional demand is the first step toward proactive self-care and burnout prevention. Ignoring it is a recipe for exhaustion, cynicism, and reduced effectiveness—essentially, losing the very MI spirit you've worked to cultivate.

Using MI Principles for Self Care Applying PACE to Yourself

Interestingly, the core principles of MI that you apply to patients can also be turned inward and applied to yourself as a form of self-care and self-compassion. Consider applying PACE to your own experience:

1. **Partnership (with Yourself):** Treat yourself as a collaborator in your own well-being, not an adversary.

Acknowledge your needs and work *with* yourself to find sustainable ways to manage stress and recharge. Are you listening to your own internal cues about needing rest or support?

2. **Acceptance (of Yourself):**
    - **Absolute Worth:** Recognize your inherent value as a person and a professional, separate from patient outcomes or daily successes and failures. You don't have to be perfect.
    - **Accurate Empathy (Self-Empathy):** Acknowledge your own feelings—frustration, fatigue, satisfaction, disappointment—without judgment. Try to understand your reactions in the context of the demanding work you do. *"It's understandable that I felt frustrated after that difficult conversation."*
    - **Autonomy Support (Self-Autonomy):** Recognize your right to set boundaries to protect your well-being (e.g., taking breaks, saying no to extra commitments when overloaded, leaving work at work as much as possible).
    - **Affirmation (Self-Affirmation):** Acknowledge your efforts, skills, and positive intentions. Notice what you *did* well, even in challenging situations. *"I handled that moment of discord calmly." "I made a real effort to understand that patient's perspective."*

3. **Compassion (Self-Compassion):** Actively promote your *own* welfare. Treat yourself with the same

kindness and understanding you would offer a respected colleague or friend facing similar challenges. Ask yourself: "What do I need right now to feel supported or replenished?" Then, act on it. This isn't selfish; it's necessary for sustained effectiveness.

4. **Evocation (of Your Strengths/Values):** Remind yourself of your own reasons for being a nurse. Connect with your core values that brought you to this profession. Draw upon your existing strengths and coping skills. What resources (internal or external) can you access when feeling depleted?

Applying MI principles inward helps counter the self-criticism and perfectionism that often contribute to burnout. It fosters a more sustainable, self-supportive internal stance.

Reflective Practice Learning from patient interactions

Motivational Interviewing is a skill that grows with practice and reflection. You won't always get it right, and every patient interaction offers potential learning. **Reflective practice** is the process of intentionally thinking about your experiences to learn from them and improve your skills and understanding. It moves beyond just *doing* MI to *thinking about* how you're doing it.

This doesn't need to be a formal, time-consuming process. It can involve brief moments of conscious reflection:

- **After a Challenging Interaction:** Take 60 seconds to ask yourself:
    - "What was the patient's perspective?"
    - "What MI skills did I use?"

- "How did the patient respond?"
- "Where did I notice change talk or sustain talk?"
- "Did I feel any discord? If so, what might have contributed to it from my end?"
- "What did I do well in that conversation?"
- "What is one thing I might try differently next time in a similar situation?"

- **Reviewing Your Day or Week:** Spend a few minutes thinking about patterns:
    - "What kinds of conversations felt most effective or energizing?"
    - "Where did I feel most stuck or frustrated?"
    - "Am I consistently using certain MI skills more than others? (e.g., Am I asking enough open questions? Am I reflecting enough?)"
    - "How well am I embodying the MI spirit?"

Keeping a Brief Reflective Journal (Optional): Some find it helpful to occasionally jot down notes about specific interactions—what happened, how they responded, what they learned. This can solidify learning and track progress over time.

Benefits of Reflective Practice:

- **Skill Development:** Consciously analyzing your practice helps refine your MI skills.

- **Increased Self-Awareness:** Understand your own communication patterns, biases, and triggers.

- **Problem-Solving:** Identify recurring challenges and brainstorm new approaches.

- **Reduced Burnout:** Processing difficult interactions reflectively can prevent negative experiences from accumulating unprocessed.

- **Reinforced Learning:** Actively thinking about MI concepts strengthens your understanding and integration.

Reflective practice turns everyday experiences into learning opportunities, fostering continuous growth and helping you stay engaged and effective.

Finding Support Peers mentors further training You dont have to do it alone

Learning and sustaining MI practice is much easier with support. Isolation can breed discouragement and burnout. Seek out connections and resources:

1. **Peer Support/Consultation:** Talk with trusted nursing colleagues who are also interested in or practicing MI. Share experiences (while maintaining patient confidentiality), discuss challenges, offer encouragement, and brainstorm strategies together. Even informal conversations can be highly beneficial. Some workplaces might facilitate peer support groups or case consultations.

2. **Mentorship/Supervision:** If possible, seek guidance from a more experienced MI practitioner or supervisor. A mentor can provide feedback (perhaps

by reviewing recorded sessions if feasible and ethically appropriate), offer insights, and help you navigate complex situations.

3. **Further Training/Workshops:** Attending booster sessions, advanced MI workshops, or topic-specific trainings (e.g., MI for chronic pain, MI in groups) can deepen your skills, introduce new perspectives, and reignite your enthusiasm. Look for opportunities offered by your institution or reputable MI training organizations.

4. **Online Resources and Communities:** Many online forums, websites, and resources are dedicated to MI (e.g., MINT - Motivational Interviewing Network of Trainers website, though be mindful of seeking practical resources over purely academic ones). These can provide articles, videos, and connections with other practitioners.

5. **Team Huddles:** Use brief team meetings or huddles to discuss challenging behavior change scenarios from an MI perspective, fostering shared learning and support within your immediate work group.

Actively seeking support normalizes challenges, provides fresh perspectives, builds skills, and reminds you that you are part of a larger community striving to communicate more effectively and compassionately.

Celebrating Successes Yours and Your Patients Acknowledge the wins big and small

In the face of daily challenges and slow progress, it's easy to focus on what's *not* working. Counteract this negativity bias by consciously acknowledging and celebrating successes—both yours and your patients'.

- **Notice Patient Progress:** Recognize and affirm any positive steps your patients take, no matter how small. Share these successes (appropriately anonymized) with supportive colleagues. Seeing patients make progress, even incremental progress, is a powerful motivator.

- **Acknowledge Your Skillful Moments:** When you handle a conversation well, use a reflection effectively, or successfully roll with discord, give yourself credit! Note these moments in your reflective practice. Recognizing your own growing competence builds confidence and satisfaction.

- **Focus on the Process, Not Just Outcomes:** Sometimes success isn't about the patient making a dramatic change immediately. Success can be building better rapport, helping a patient feel understood for the first time, facilitating their exploration of ambivalence, or collaboratively creating one small plan. Celebrate these process wins.

- **Share Positive Stories:** In team meetings or peer discussions, make space for sharing positive experiences and examples of MI making a difference. This builds collective morale and reinforces the value of the approach.

Actively looking for and celebrating successes helps maintain a positive perspective, counteracts fatigue, and reinforces the rewarding aspects of this work.

Nursing Focus Maintaining enthusiasm and effectiveness using MI long term

Sustaining MI practice over a nursing career requires intentionality. It's not a one-time training but an ongoing commitment to skillful and compassionate communication. Key strategies for long-term success include:

- **Integrate, Don't Add:** Focus on weaving MI into your existing workflow, not seeing it as a separate burden. Use those fly-bys and high-yield moments.
- **Stay Curious:** Maintain genuine curiosity about your patients' perspectives. Curiosity fuels empathy and keeps interactions fresh.
- **Practice Self-Compassion Regularly:** Apply PACE principles inwardly. Be kind to yourself, especially on difficult days.
- **Make Reflection a Habit:** Build brief moments of reflection into your routine to continuously learn and grow.
- **Seek Connection:** Combat isolation by connecting with peers, mentors, or MI learning communities.
- **Manage Expectations:** Accept that change is often slow and non-linear. Focus on facilitating the process and celebrating small steps.
- **Reconnect with Your "Why":** Regularly remind yourself of your core nursing values and the reasons you chose this profession. MI is a powerful tool for living out those values.

- **Set Boundaries:** Protect your time and energy to prevent exhaustion. Learn to say no when needed.

By tending to both your skills and your own well-being, you can maintain the enthusiasm and effectiveness needed to use MI as a powerful tool for supporting your patients and finding deeper satisfaction in your nursing practice for years to come.

Staying the Course Key Takeaways

- Supporting behavior change involves significant **emotional labor**; acknowledging this is key to preventing burnout.

- Apply MI principles (**PACE**) inwardly for **self-care**: partner with yourself, accept your limitations with empathy, act with self-compassion, and evoke your own strengths and values.

- Engage in **reflective practice** by intentionally thinking about interactions to learn, refine skills, and increase self-awareness.

- Combat isolation by actively seeking **support** from peers, mentors, further training, and online communities.

- Consciously **celebrate successes**—both patient progress (small wins count!) and your own skillful moments—to maintain a positive perspective.

- Long-term sustainability involves integrating MI into workflow, staying curious, practicing self-compassion, reflecting regularly, seeking connection, managing expectations, reconnecting with values, and setting boundaries.

(Transition to Conclusion) You have journeyed through the spirit, skills, applications, and sustainability of Motivational Interviewing in nursing. We've explored how this approach can transform conversations and empower patients. Now, let's draw together the threads and reflect on the broader impact of embracing MI as a fundamental aspect of compassionate and effective nursing care.

Conclusion: Empowering Patients, Empowering Yourself

We began this guide by acknowledging a common frustration in nursing—the challenge of helping patients make difficult but necessary changes to improve their health. We recognized that simply providing expert advice often isn't enough. We then introduced Motivational Interviewing not as another complex technique to be mastered, but as a fundamental shift in communication—a way of being *with* patients that honors their autonomy, evokes their own motivation, and fosters a collaborative partnership.

Throughout these chapters, we've moved from the foundational **Spirit of MI** (Partnership, Acceptance, Compassion, Evocation) and its guiding principles, to mastering the practical **OARS skills** (Open questions, Affirmations, Reflections, Summaries). We learned to tune our ears to **change talk**, the patient's own arguments for change, and how to respond effectively using **EARS** (Elaborate, Affirm, Reflect, Summarize). We explored the normalcy of **ambivalence** and learned strategies for **rolling with discord** rather than arguing against it. We addressed the necessity of information exchange through the collaborative **Elicit-Provide-Elicit** framework. We then moved into action, discussing how to guide patients through **collaborative planning** using **SMART(er)** goals and anticipating barriers. We saw MI **in motion** through common nursing scenarios, demonstrating its applicability even in brief encounters. We tackled the crucial issue of **integrating MI into busy workflows** and, finally, addressed the importance of **sustaining your practice** through self-care and reflection.

Recap of Key Benefits Increased engagement improved adherence stronger rapport greater job satisfaction

Why undertake this shift in communication? The benefits extend to both your patients and yourself:

- **For Patients:**
    - **Increased Engagement:** Patients who feel heard, understood, and respected are more likely to actively participate in their own care.
    - **Improved Adherence:** By connecting health behaviors to the patient's own values and goals, MI can lead to more sustained adherence to treatment plans and lifestyle changes compared to directive approaches.
    - **Greater Empowerment:** MI helps patients discover their own reasons, resources, and confidence for change, fostering a sense of agency and self-efficacy.

- o **Reduced Resistance:** A collaborative approach minimizes discord, making potentially difficult conversations smoother.

- **For You, the Nurse:**
  - o **Stronger Rapport:** MI builds trust and strengthens the therapeutic relationship, making interactions more positive.
  - o **Increased Effectiveness:** Seeing patients make genuine progress based on their own motivation is professionally rewarding.
  - o **Reduced Frustration:** Avoiding arguments and power struggles can make challenging conversations less stressful.
  - o **Greater Job Satisfaction:** Feeling more effective, connected to patients, and aligned with compassionate nursing values can significantly enhance job satisfaction and potentially reduce burnout.

The Long View MI as a fundamental communication skill for compassionate effective nursing

Motivational Interviewing is more than a set of techniques for behavior change. It is a communication style deeply rooted in respect, empathy, and collaboration—hallmarks of excellent nursing care. It provides a practical framework for enacting patient-centeredness in everyday interactions. While initially developed for specific counseling contexts, its principles and skills offer a way to enhance communication across the entire spectrum of nursing practice.

Learning MI is indeed a journey, not a destination. It requires ongoing practice, reflection, and a willingness to sometimes stumble and try again. But the potential rewards—more engaged patients, improved health outcomes, and a more satisfying professional experience for you—make it a journey well worth taking. It equips you not just to treat illness, but to truly partner with people as they navigate the complex path toward better health and well-being.

A Final Encouragement

As you continue to integrate these principles and skills into your practice, be patient with yourself. Celebrate the small successes. Seek support when you need it. Trust in the power of genuine listening and collaboration. By embracing the spirit and practice of Motivational Interviewing, you not only empower your patients to find their own path to change, but you also empower yourself to be a more effective, compassionate, and resilient nurse. You are making a difference, one conversation at a time.

Chapter 10: Case Studies Applying MI Across Nursing Settings

The preceding chapters laid out the framework—the spirit, the principles, the skills, the strategies for handling specific situations like planning or information exchange. But the real test, and the real learning, often comes from seeing these ideas put into practice in the varied and often unpredictable situations nurses encounter daily. This chapter presents ten case studies drawn from diverse nursing settings. Each case illustrates how a nurse integrated Motivational Interviewing principles and techniques into their interaction with a patient facing a common health behavior challenge. Pay attention to the nurse's choices—the questions asked, the reflections offered, the way information is shared, how discord is handled, and how collaboration is maintained. These are not meant as perfect examples, but as realistic illustrations of MI in motion.

Case Study 1 Primary Care Addressing HbA1c with Mr Chen Revisited

- **Setting:** Busy primary care clinic.
- **Nurse:** Davis, RN, BSN.
- **Patient:** Mr. Chen, 58, with Type 2 diabetes and hypertension, presenting with an elevated HbA1c of 9.2%. (Referenced in earlier chapters).
- **Focus:** Exploring reasons for elevated A1c, fostering collaboration around management.

Interaction:

(Recall from Chapter 2, Nurse Davis starts with an open question about Mr. Chen's thoughts on the A1c result, reflecting his challenges and feelings of discouragement related to work stress and perceived failure).

Nurse Davis: ... "**Okay, so we have this situation where the medication helps with focus and family relationships** [referring back to earlier change talk not detailed here], **but the side effects like weight gain and drowsiness are a major problem for you.** [Reflecting previously discussed medication issues, not the focus of *this* interaction but part of the overall picture]. **Thinking specifically about managing the blood sugars day-to-day, what feels like the biggest hurdle right now?**" (**Summary** of a related issue, **Open Question** refocusing on diabetes self-management).

Mr. Chen: "Honestly? It's the diet. Especially lunches at work. Everyone orders takeout—pizza, Chinese... it's fast and easy. Packing a lunch feels like another chore."

Nurse Davis: "**So, convenience and fitting in with coworkers makes takeout appealing at lunch, while packing a healthier lunch feels like added work on top of everything else.**" (**Complex Reflection** capturing the push-pull).

Mr. Chen: "Exactly. And then I feel guilty, so sometimes I just skip checking my sugar later."

Nurse Davis: "**The guilt about lunch choices sometimes leads to avoiding the blood sugar check altogether.**" (**Reflection** linking behaviors). "**That makes sense—it's tough to face the number when you suspect it might not be what you want.**" (**Empathy/Normalizing**). "**You know, you're really good at identifying these patterns.**"

(**Affirmation**). "**Given that work lunches are a major challenge, what *potential* small change—even one day a week—might feel possible regarding lunch?**" (**Open Question** exploring small steps/Ability).

Mr. Chen: "Maybe... maybe I could pack a lunch just on Mondays? Start of the week?" (**Activation/Ability**).

Nurse Davis: "**Packing a lunch just on Mondays to start the week off.**" (**Reflection**). "**How confident do you feel about trying that for the next, say, two weeks? Scale of 0 to 10?**" (**Open Question** - assessing confidence).

Mr. Chen: "Maybe a 6 or 7. It's just one day."

Nurse Davis: "**A 6 or 7. So fairly confident, because it's just one day.**" (**Reflection**). "**What keeps it from being higher? What might get in the way?**" (**Open Question** exploring barriers).

Mr. Chen: "Forgetting to make it the night before, mostly."

Nurse Davis: "**Ah, so remembering Sunday night would be key.**" (**Reflection**). "**How could you remind yourself?**" (**Open Question** - eliciting solution).

Mr. Chen: "Put a note on the fridge, I guess."

Analysis: Nurse Davis uses OARS consistently—open questions to explore barriers and solutions, reflections to ensure understanding and explore ambivalence, and affirmations to build confidence. She avoids the righting reflex (no lecturing about takeout), focuses on a specific barrier identified by Mr. Chen (work lunches), and guides him toward a small, achievable, self-generated plan (pack lunch Mondays, use a reminder note). She checks confidence to ensure the plan is realistic.

Case Study 2 Community Health Smoking Cessation with Maria Revisited

- **Setting:** Home visit by community health nurse.
- **Nurse:** Sarah, RN.
- **Patient:** Maria, 35, mother of two, smokes ~1 pack/day, feels overwhelmed but wants to quit "someday." (Referenced in Chapter 3).
- **Focus:** Exploring ambivalence about smoking, identifying potential small steps.

Interaction:

(Recall from Chapter 3, Sarah uses reflections to explore Maria's desire to quit vs. reliance on smoking for coping. Maria identifies cost and health worries as reasons to quit. Sarah affirms Maria's past attempt and explores what was learned. Maria expresses willingness to consider making the car smoke-free).

Sarah: "**Okay, so making the car smoke-free is something you're considering.**" (**Reflection** - Activation). "**What would be the best things about doing that?**" (**Open Question** - eliciting Reasons/benefits of the *specific step*).

Maria: "Well, the kids wouldn't complain about the smell anymore. And maybe... maybe it would help me cut down overall without feeling like I'm totally deprived?"

Sarah: "**So, potential benefits are happier kids regarding the smell, and it might be a way to reduce your smoking without the pressure of full quitting right now.**" (**Summary** of benefits). **"That sounds like a thoughtful approach."** (**Affirmation**).

Maria: "But what about when I get really stressed driving in traffic?"

Sarah: **"Good point—driving stress is a major trigger for you."** (**Reflection** identifying barrier). **"If you decided *not* to smoke in the car, what else could you possibly do during those stressful driving moments?"** (**Open Question** - brainstorming alternatives).

Maria: "Chew gum? Listen to loud music? I don't know."

Sarah: **"Chewing gum and turning up music are a couple of ideas."** (**Reflection**). **"Of those, or perhaps something else, what seems like the most appealing or realistic option to try?"** (**Open Question** - clarifying preferred strategy).

Maria: "Maybe the music. I could make a playlist."

Sarah: **"Making a specific 'stressful commute' playlist could be your go-to strategy."** (**Reflection**). **"So, the possible plan taking shape is: Designate the car as smoke-free, and have a music playlist ready for stressful driving moments."** (**Summary**). **"How does that sit with you as an experiment for, say, the next week?"** (**Open Question** - checking readiness/commitment).

Maria: "An experiment... yeah, maybe I could try it for a week. See what happens." (**Activation/Commitment** to experiment).

Analysis: Sarah continues to use OARS, particularly reflections and open questions. She helps Maria articulate the benefits of the specific step (car smoke-free), anticipates barriers (stressful driving), facilitates brainstorming of alternative coping strategies, and frames the plan as an "experiment," which can feel less daunting than a permanent commitment. She supports Maria's autonomy throughout.

Case Study 3 Mental Health Inpatient Engaging Liam in Activity Revisited

- **Setting:** Inpatient mental health unit.
- **Nurse:** Chen, RN.
- **Patient:** Liam, 28, experiencing depression, withdrawn, declines group therapy. (Referenced in Chapter 7).
- **Focus:** Building rapport, finding one small positive action Liam is willing to take.

Interaction:

(Recall from Chapter 7, Chen uses empathy and reflections to acknowledge Liam's hopelessness and resistance to group. He affirms Liam's resilience and explores alternative activities. Liam identifies listening to music as something that sometimes helps "a little.")

Chen: "**Music helps a bit sometimes.**" (**Reflection**). "**Would you be open to making sure you have access to your music player and headphones today, maybe aiming to listen for at least 15-20 minutes?**" (**Elicit** permission/Activation for a small, patient-identified step).

Liam: (Slight hesitation) "I guess."

Chen: "**It sounds like you're willing to give it a try.**" (**Reflection** - Activation). "**Where is your music player now? Do you need help finding it or making sure it's charged?**" (**Open Question** - facilitating the action).

Liam: "Think it's in my drawer. Probably needs charging."

Chen: "**Okay. So, a concrete first step is finding it and getting it charged.**" (**Reflection** - breaking down the action). "**Is that something you feel up for doing right now, or would you like me to hang onto it at the nurses' station to charge?**" (**Open Question** offering support/choice).

Liam: "You can charge it."

Chen: "**Happy to.** (Affirmation/Partnership). **Once it's charged, when might be a good time for you to try listening for those 15-20 minutes? Maybe this afternoon?**" (**Open Question** - planning specifics).

Liam: "Maybe."

Chen: "**Okay. How about I bring it back to you around 2 pm, fully charged, and you can decide then if it feels like the right time?**" (**Summarizing plan**, respecting autonomy/timing).

Liam: (Nods).

Analysis: Chen accepts Liam's minimal engagement without pushing. He focuses on the one small positive Liam identified (music). He breaks the action down into even smaller steps (find player, charge it). He offers concrete help (charging it), removing a potential barrier. He plans the next step collaboratively but leaves the final decision about *when* to listen up to Liam, fully respecting his autonomy while gently encouraging movement. The immediate goal isn't deep engagement, but facilitating one small, patient-chosen positive behavior.

Case Study 4 Chronic Illness COPD Self-Management with Mrs Diaz Revisited

- **Setting:** Pulmonary clinic follow-up.
- **Nurse:** Simone, NP.
- **Patient:** Mrs. Diaz, 72, with COPD, sometimes forgets controller inhaler. (Referenced in Chapter 7).
- **Focus:** Following up on previous plan, exploring ongoing self-management.

Interaction:

Simone: "Mrs. Diaz, last time we met, you decided to try keeping your purple controller inhaler on your nightstand to help remember the evening dose. **How has that strategy been working out for you over the past few weeks?**" (**Open Question** - checking on previous plan).

Mrs. Diaz: "Oh, much better! It's right there, I see it with my pills. I think I've only missed it once or twice when I fell asleep early."

Simone: "**That's wonderful! Moving it to the nightstand has made a big difference in remembering that evening dose.**" (**Affirmation**). "**And you've identified that falling asleep early is still an occasional challenge.**" (**Reflection** - acknowledging ongoing minor barrier).

Mrs. Diaz: "Yes, but it's much improved."

Simone: "**That's excellent progress.**" (**Affirmation**). "**Thinking about managing your COPD overall, besides the inhalers, what else feels important to you right now? Perhaps activity levels, or managing flare-ups?**" (**Open Question** - broadening focus/exploring priorities).

Mrs. Diaz: "Well, I still get so breathless when I walk up the stairs. I wish I could do that easier." (**Change Talk - Desire/Reason**).

Simone: "**Feeling less breathless on the stairs is something you really want.**" (**Reflection** - Desire). "**What have you tried, or what have you considered, that might help with managing breathlessness during activities like stair climbing?**" (**Open Question** - exploring strategies/Ability).

Mrs. Diaz: "The pulmonary rehab people taught me pursed-lip breathing, but I forget to use it."

Simone: "**So you have a tool—pursed-lip breathing—that you know could help, but remembering to use it in the moment is the tricky part.**" (**Reflection** summarizing the specific challenge). "**What might remind you or make it easier to use that technique right when you approach the stairs?**" (**Open Question** - eliciting solutions).

Mrs. Diaz: "Maybe... put a little sticky note at the bottom of the stairs? Just the word 'Breathe'?"

Simone: "**A visual cue like a 'Breathe' note at the bottom of the stairs.**" (**Reflection**). "**That's a creative idea.**" (**Affirmation**). "**How confident are you that seeing that note would help you remember to use the pursed-lip breathing?**" (**Open Question** - checking confidence).

Analysis: Simone starts by following up on the previous plan, affirming success. She then uses an open question to explore other patient priorities. She reflects Mrs. Diaz's desire (less breathlessness), explores existing knowledge/strategies (pursed-lip breathing), identifies the specific barrier (remembering to use it), and guides Mrs. Diaz to a self-generated, concrete reminder strategy (sticky note). She maintains partnership throughout.

Case Study 5 Emergency Department Brief Intervention for Alcohol Use

- **Setting:** Busy Emergency Department.
- **Nurse:** Ben, RN.
- **Patient:** Mark, 30, presenting with a minor wrist injury after falling; smells of alcohol, admits to drinking "a few beers" before the fall. Screening tool suggests hazardous drinking pattern.
- **Focus:** Briefly raising awareness about alcohol use and potential risks, assessing readiness for change. (Goal is brief intervention, not full treatment).

Interaction:

Ben: "Mark, thanks for being honest about having a few beers before the fall. We also did this brief questionnaire about alcohol use, which suggests your current level of drinking might put you at increased risk for health problems or injuries like this one down the road. **What are your thoughts on that?**" (**Linking behavior to risk neutrally**, **Elicit** - reaction).

Mark: "Nah, I'm fine. I just lost my balance. Everyone drinks."

Ben: "**So from your perspective, the fall was just an accident, not really related to the drinking, and your current level feels normal to you.**" (**Reflection** of sustain talk/patient perspective). "**And it's true, many people drink alcohol.**" (**Agreeing with a twist** - partial agreement). "**At the same time, the screening suggests potential risks.** (Restating concern neutrally). **On a scale of 0 to 10, where 0 is not at all important and 10 is extremely important, how important would you say it is for you to keep your drinking at a level that avoids future health risks or injuries?**" (**Open Question** - assessing importance/Need using scaling).

Mark: "Maybe a 4 or 5? I mean, I don't *want* to get hurt again." (**Some Need/Reason** emerges).

Ben: "**So, a 4 or 5. It's definitely on your radar – avoiding future injuries is important to you.**" (**Reflection** highlighting the change talk aspect). "**What makes it a 4 or 5, rather than a 0 or 1?**" (**Open Question** - eliciting reasons for importance).

Mark: "Like I said, I don't want to end up back here. And my girlfriend gives me grief about it sometimes."

Ben: "**So avoiding future ED visits and maybe having things smoother with your girlfriend are reasons why managing your drinking has some importance for you.**" (**Summary** of Reasons). "**Okay. Thanks for talking about this. Since it has *some* importance, would you be open to looking at this information card? It just shows what lower-risk drinking limits generally look like and has** some resources if you ever *did* want to cut back." (**Affirmation**, **Elicit** permission to provide info using EPE).

Mark: "Uh, sure, I guess I can take it."

Ben: "(Hands card) **Great. Take a look whenever you like. What questions do you have right now?**" (**Provide**, **Elicit** reaction/questions).

Analysis: Ben keeps the intervention brief and focused. He uses reflections to acknowledge Mark's initial dismissal (rolling with discord). He uses scaling questions to gently probe importance (Need) without being confrontational. He reflects the change talk that emerges ("avoiding injuries," "smoother with girlfriend"). He uses EPE to offer information respectfully (asks permission, provides neutrally, asks for reaction). The goal isn't immediate change, but raising awareness, planting a seed, and offering resources, all within the ED's time constraints.

Case Study 6 Pediatric Clinic Discussing Vaccinations with Hesitant Parent

- **Setting:** Pediatric primary care clinic.
- **Nurse:** Linda, LPN.
- **Patient/Client:** Ms. Evans, mother of 1-year-old Maya, expressing hesitation about MMR vaccine.
- **Focus:** Exploring concerns, providing information using EPE, respecting parental autonomy.

Interaction:

Linda: "Ms. Evans, according to Maya's schedule, she's due for her MMR vaccine today. **What thoughts or questions do you have about the MMR vaccine?**" (**Stating recommendation neutrally, Open Question** exploring perspective).

Ms. Evans: "I don't know... I've read some things online about it... links to autism? It makes me nervous."

Linda: "**It sounds like you've come across some information online that's made you feel nervous, specifically about a possible link between the MMR vaccine and autism.**" (**Reflection** capturing concern/source).

Ms. Evans: "Yes. I just want to do what's best for Maya."

Linda: "**Wanting the very best for Maya is your top priority.**" (**Affirmation** of value/intention). "**You're being a careful parent by looking into these things.**" (**Affirmation**). "**Would you be open to hearing about the scientific research that has looked very closely at that specific concern?**" (**Elicit** permission to provide info).

Ms. Evans: "Okay, yes. What does the research say?"

Linda: "**Multiple large-scale, carefully conducted scientific studies involving hundreds of thousands of children across different countries have specifically investigated this question.** (Provide - context). **These studies have consistently shown *no link* between the MMR vaccine and autism.** (Provide - neutral summary of findings). **The original study that suggested a link back in the late 90s was found to have serious flaws and was retracted by the journal that published it.** (Provide - additional context). **Major health organizations worldwide,** based on this extensive evidence, strongly recommend the MMR vaccine as safe and effective protection against measles, mumps, and rubella, which can be serious diseases." (Provide - recommendation based on evidence).

Linda: "**What are your thoughts or reactions hearing that information?**" (**Elicit** - reaction/understanding).

Ms. Evans: "So... all those big studies found nothing? And the first one was wrong?"

Linda: "**That's correct. The overwhelming scientific consensus, based on studies of hundreds of thousands of children, is that there is no connection between the MMR vaccine and autism.**" (**Reflection/Provide** - reinforcing key message). "**How does that information sit with you now, compared to what you read online?**" (**Open Question** exploring impact).

Ms. Evans: "It's... confusing. But maybe the websites I saw weren't reliable. The thought of measles scares me too." (**Ambivalence/Change Talk - Reason**).

Linda: "**So you're weighing the reassurance from the large scientific studies against the scary things you read online, and also considering the real risks of diseases like measles.**" (**Double-Sided Reflection**). "**Given all that, what feels like the right decision for Maya today regarding the MMR vaccine? It's absolutely your choice.**" (**Open Question** inviting decision, **Emphasizing Autonomy**).

Analysis: Linda starts by eliciting concerns non-judgmentally. She reflects and affirms the parent's core motivation (wanting best for child). She uses EPE effectively—asking permission, providing clear, neutral summaries of scientific consensus, and then eliciting the parent's reaction and integration of the information. She acknowledges the conflicting information and reflects the remaining ambivalence before respectfully asking for a decision while affirming autonomy.

Case Study 7 Oncology Clinic Addressing Treatment Side Effects Nausea

- **Setting:** Outpatient oncology clinic.
- **Nurse:** Fatima, RN, OCN.
- **Patient:** Mr. Lee, 62, undergoing chemotherapy, reporting significant nausea affecting his quality of life.
- **Focus:** Exploring the impact of nausea, collaborating on management strategies.

Interaction:

Fatima: "Mr. Lee, you mentioned on the phone that the nausea has been quite bad with this last cycle. **Tell me more about how it's been affecting you day-to-day.**" (**Open Question** exploring impact).

Mr. Lee: "It's awful. I feel sick all the time. Don't want to eat. Don't want to do anything. Just lie around."

Fatima: "**So the nausea is really pervasive, wiping out your appetite and energy, and basically putting your life on hold.**" (**Complex Reflection** capturing depth of impact).

Mr. Lee: "Exactly. What's the point of fighting the cancer if I feel this miserable?" (**Expression of despair/questioning value**).

Fatima: "**It sounds incredibly discouraging, to the point where the side effects make you question if the treatment itself is worth it.**" (**Reflection** validating feeling/dilemma). "That must be a very tough place to be." (**Empathy**). "You've shown amazing strength getting through these treatments so far." (**Affirmation**).

Mr. Lee: "I try."

Fatima: "**You absolutely do.** (Affirmation). **We definitely want to manage this nausea better so you don't feel so miserable.** (Partnership/Goal). **You're already taking the anti-nausea pills we prescribed. How consistently have you been taking them?**" (**Open Question** checking adherence).

Mr. Lee: "I take them when I feel really sick."

Fatima: "**So you tend to take them *reactively*, once the nausea is already bad.**" (**Reflection**). "Would you be open to hearing how these particular medications often work best?" (**Elicit** permission - EPE).

Mr. Lee: "Sure."

Fatima: "**These anti-nausea medications often work much better at *preventing* nausea than at stopping it once it's severe.** (Provide - neutral info). **Taking them on a regular schedule, even if you're not feeling sick at that exact moment, can often keep the nausea from getting bad in the first place.**" (Provide - rationale). "**What are your thoughts about trying that—taking them on a set schedule for the first few days after chemo, regardless of how you feel?**" (**Elicit** - reaction/inviting collaboration on strategy).

Mr. Lee: "You mean, take them even if I feel okay?"

Fatima: "**Exactly, taking them regularly, say every 8 hours for the first 3 days, as a preventative measure.**" (**Clarifying Provide**). "How does that idea strike you?" (**Elicit** - reaction).

Mr. Lee: "I guess it makes sense. If it could stop it before it starts... I'd **be willing to try** anything at this point." (**Reason/Activation**).

Analysis: Fatima uses reflections and empathy extensively to validate Mr. Lee's profound distress. She affirms his strength before exploring the current strategy. She uses EPE to explain the rationale for scheduled vs. PRN antiemetics. She presents the new strategy as an option ("What are your thoughts about trying...") and reflects his willingness to try, confirming the collaborative plan.

Case Study 8 Surgical Unit Pre op Anxiety Reduction

- **Setting:** Pre-operative holding area.
- **Nurse:** Carlos, RN.
- **Patient:** Ms. Garcia, 45, scheduled for hysterectomy, appears visibly anxious.
- **Focus:** Acknowledging anxiety, exploring coping, offering brief relaxation strategy.

Interaction:

Carlos: "Ms. Garcia, I'm Carlos, your nurse helping get you ready for surgery. I notice you seem quite anxious this morning. **What's going through your mind right now?**" (**Observation, Empathy, Open Question**).

Ms. Garcia: (Tearfully) "I'm just so scared. What if something goes wrong? I've never had major surgery."

Carlos: "**It sounds like the fear of the unknown and potential complications is really strong for you, especially since this is your first major surgery.**" (**Complex Reflection** capturing fear/reason). "**It's completely normal to feel scared before an operation like this.**" (**Normalizing**).

Ms. Garcia: "My hands are shaking."

Carlos: "**You're feeling the anxiety physically in your body right now.**" (**Reflection**). "**You've been incredibly brave getting to this point.**" (**Affirmation**). "**What usually helps you cope when you feel anxious or scared?**" (**Open Question** exploring existing coping skills).

Ms. Garcia: "Sometimes listening to music helps calm me down. Or just deep breaths."

Carlos: "**So you already have some tools that work for you – music and deep breathing.**" (**Reflection/Affirmation** of strengths). "**Would you be open to trying just a minute or two of slow, deep breathing right now? Sometimes focusing on the breath can help calm those physical sensations, even just a little.**" (**Linking to patient's idea, Elicit** permission - EPE structure for suggesting strategy).

Ms. Garcia: "Okay. I can try."

Carlos: "**Great.** (Guides briefly). **Just breathing slowly in through your nose… and gently out through your mouth… letting your belly rise and fall… Just focusing on the sensation of the breath..." (**Provide** - guiding technique). *(After a minute)* "**How does that feel now?**" (**Elicit** - reaction).

Ms. Garcia: "A little better. Still nervous, but... maybe not shaking as much."

Carlos: "**So taking those few slow breaths helped calm the physical feelings a bit, even though the worry is still there.**" (**Reflection**). "That's good information. You can use that technique anytime you feel the anxiety rising while you're waiting." (**Reinforcing strategy/Supporting Self-Efficacy**).

Analysis: Carlos immediately addresses the observed anxiety with empathy and an open question. He normalizes her fear and reflects her specific concerns. He evokes her existing coping skills and affirms them. He then builds on *her* suggestion (deep breaths), asks permission to guide her, provides brief instruction, and elicits feedback. He supports her self-efficacy by reminding her she can use this tool herself.

Case Study 9 Home Health Wound Care Adherence

- **Setting:** Patient's home.
- **Nurse:** Diane, RN, WOCN.
- **Patient:** Mr. Evans, 78, lives alone, has a chronic venous leg ulcer requiring daily dressing changes; struggles with consistency.
- **Focus:** Exploring barriers to dressing changes, problem-solving collaboratively.

Interaction:

Diane: "Mr. Evans, looking at your leg today, the wound looks okay, but the edges seem a bit macerated, suggesting the dressing might not be getting changed quite daily. **How has it been going with doing the dressing changes each day?**" (**Observation linked to behavior**, **Open Question**).

Mr. Evans: "Oh, Diane, it's just so hard. Bending over hurts my back. And my fingers are stiff these days. Sometimes I just… skip it."

Diane: "**So the physical difficulty—bending that hurts your back and stiff fingers—makes the daily dressing change a real chore, sometimes leading you to skip it altogether.**" (**Complex Reflection** summarizing barriers).

Mr. Evans: "Yes. I know I should do it…" (**Change talk - Need**, but weak).

Diane: "**Part of you knows it's important for healing.**" (**Reflection** of change talk). "**And it's completely understandable that tasks become harder with back pain and stiffness.**" (Empathy/Normalizing). "**You manage so much independently here, which is really impressive.**" (Affirmation). "**Let's put our heads together. Thinking about the challenges—the bending and the finger stiffness—what potential adjustments or tools might make the process even slightly easier?**" (**Partnership**, **Open Question** inviting solutions).

Mr. Evans: "Maybe if I sat down? Put my foot up on a stool? Less bending that way."

Diane: "**Sitting down with your foot elevated on a stool could definitely reduce the bending.**" (Reflection). "That's a great idea to try." (**Affirmation**). "What about the stiff fingers part? Anything that might help with opening packages or handling the gauze?" (**Open Question** focusing on second barrier).

Mr. Evans: "My neighbor sometimes helps open jars for me... maybe... maybe she could help open the dressing packages ahead of time?"

Diane: "**Asking your neighbor for help just with opening the packages in advance.**" (**Reflection**). "**How would you feel about asking her for that specific type of help?**" (**Open Question** assessing comfort/Ability).

Mr. Evans: "She's very kind. I think she wouldn't mind just doing that."

Diane: "**Okay, so two potential strategies: Sit with your foot on a stool for the dressing change, and ask your neighbor to pre-open the packages.**" (**Summary**). "**How do these ideas sound as things to try this week?**" (**Open Question** checking commitment).

Mr. Evans: "Yes, I can try those. That might just make it manageable." (**Ability/Activation**).

Analysis: Diane avoids blame or lecture about non-adherence. She reflects Mr. Evans's specific physical barriers with empathy. She affirms his independence before inviting collaboration ("Let's put our heads together"). She guides him to brainstorm solutions for *each* identified barrier separately. She checks his comfort level with involving a neighbor. The resulting plan directly addresses his stated difficulties and comes from his own ideas.

Case Study 10 School Health Addressing Frequent Absences Related to Anxiety

- **Setting:** High school nurse's office.
- **Nurse:** Rachel, BSN, RN.
- **Patient:** Chloe, 15, frequently visits nurse's office with vague complaints (headache, stomachache) often resulting in calls home; pattern suggests underlying anxiety.
- **Focus:** Building rapport, gently exploring potential anxiety link, identifying coping strategies.

Interaction:

Rachel: "Chloe, you're back in today feeling unwell. **Tell me what's happening for you right now.**" (**Acknowledging visit, Open Question**).

Chloe: "My stomach hurts. And I feel kind of shaky."

Rachel: "**So your stomach hurts and you're feeling shaky inside.**" (**Reflection**). *(Takes vital signs, performs brief assessment - all within normal limits).* "**Physically, everything looks stable right now.**" (Sharing finding neutrally). "**I've noticed you've been coming in feeling this way fairly often lately, especially before big tests or presentations.**" (**Observation/Pattern Reflection**, gently linking to potential triggers). "**What do you make of that pattern?**" (**Open Question** inviting insight).

Chloe: (Looks down) "I don't know. Maybe I just get sick easily."

Rachel: "**That's one possibility.**" (**Reflection** accepting her view). "**Sometimes, when people have important or** stressful things coming up, their bodies react with physical feelings like stomachaches or shakiness—kind of like worry showing up physically." (**Provide** - normalizing psycho-physiological link neutrally). "**Does that sound at all familiar, or not really?**" (**Elicit** - reaction).

Chloe: (Hesitantly) "Maybe. I *do* get really stressed about tests."

Rachel: "**So you recognize that stress about tests is a big thing for you, and it's possible these physical feelings might be connected to that stress.**" (**Reflection** linking stress and physical symptoms). "**That takes self-awareness to notice.**" (**Affirmation**).

Chloe: "I hate feeling this way." (**Desire**).

Rachel: "**You really wish you didn't have to go through this.**" (**Reflection** - Desire). "**When you feel this stress or worry building up, what, if anything, sometimes helps you feel even a tiny bit better or calmer?**" (**Open Question** - exploring coping).

Chloe: "Talking to my friend helps sometimes. Or doodling in my notebook."

Rachel: "**Talking with your friend and doodling are two things already in your toolkit that can help manage the stress.**" (**Reflection/Affirmation** - strengths). "**Those are great strategies.**" (**Affirmation**). "**Thinking about next time you feel this way *before* it gets bad enough to leave class, how might you use one of those strategies—talking to your friend briefly or doing some quick doodling—right there in the classroom or hallway?**" (**Open Question** - planning preventative coping).

Analysis: Rachel avoids immediately labeling Chloe's symptoms as "just anxiety." She validates the physical feelings while gently introducing the potential stress link through observation and neutral information provision (EPE-like). She reflects Chloe's growing awareness and desire for change. She evokes Chloe's *existing* coping strategies and helps her plan how to use them proactively, empowering her to manage the feelings *before* needing to leave class. The focus is on coping and self-management, not eliminating anxiety entirely.

Lessons from the Field

These cases illustrate several recurring themes:

- MI is adaptable across diverse settings and patient situations.[1]

- Starting with **Open Questions** and **Reflective Listening** is almost always the right first step to build rapport and understand the patient's world.

- **Affirming** patient strengths, efforts, and positive intentions is crucial for building confidence.

- **Rolling with Discord** non-judgmentally keeps conversations open when disagreement or frustration arises.

- Using **EPE** ensures information is shared collaboratively and respectfully.

- Guiding patients to develop their **own plans**, starting with **small, achievable steps**, is key to fostering ownership and success.

- Even **brief interactions**, using MI strategically, can be impactful.

These examples provide a glimpse into the possibilities. As you continue your practice, you will develop your own style and discover countless ways to apply these principles to support your patients effectively.

(Transition) Having seen MI applied in these varied contexts, the journey concludes by revisiting the core benefits and encouraging your continued growth in this rewarding approach to nursing communication. The Appendices that follow offer quick references to aid your ongoing practice.

Appendices

Quick Reference Guide MI Spirit Principles

- A breakdown of the **PACE** acronym: **P**artnership, **A**cceptance (including Autonomy, Absolute Worth, Accurate Empathy, Affirmation), **C**ompassion, **E**vocation, with brief descriptions of each element in nursing terms.

- A summary of the four guiding **Principles**: Expressing Empathy, Developing Discrepancy, Rolling with Resistance/Discord, Supporting Self-Efficacy, with key action points for each.

- Perhaps a few bullet points contrasting an MI approach with a more directive approach.

Quick Reference Guide OARS Sentence Starters

- **Open Questions:** Lists of starting phrases like "How...", "What...", "Tell me about...", "Describe...", "In what ways...". Examples tailored to assessment, exploring ambivalence, and planning.

- **Affirmations:** Examples focusing on effort, strengths, intentions, and values. Phrasing like "You really...", "It took courage to...", "You're someone who...".

- **Reflections:** Stems like "It sounds like...", "You're feeling...", "So you...", "It seems...", with examples of simple, complex, and double-sided reflections.

- **Summaries:** Starting phrases for collecting, linking, or transitional summaries, such as "So let me see if I've got this right...", "That connects back to...", "So, to recap...".

Quick Reference Guide Elicit Provide Elicit Checklist

- **Elicit (Step 1):** Checkbox items like "Assessed patient's current knowledge?" "Asked permission to share information?" with sample phrasing.
- **Provide (Step 2):** Reminders like "Information clear and concise?" "Neutral language used?" "Avoided jargon?" "Offered in small chunks?".
- **Elicit (Step 3):** Checkbox items like "Asked for patient's reaction/understanding?" "Used an open question (e.g., 'What are your thoughts on that?')" "Checked for questions?".
- Possibly a very brief example dialogue illustrating the flow.

Sample Phrasing for Common Nursing Situations

- Addressing medication non-adherence.
- Opening a conversation about lifestyle changes (smoking, diet, exercise).
- Responding to expressions of low motivation or hopelessness.
- Discussing abnormal lab results or vital signs.
- Handling missed appointments.

- Responding to patient complaints or frustration.
- Initiating goal setting or action planning.

References

1. Bergh, H., Johansson, K. and Hildingh, C. (2018) 'Motivational interviewing in health promotion: Experiences among nurses and patients in primary healthcare', *Primary Health Care Research & Development*, 19(2), pp. 155-166.

2. Bohman, A., Rasmussen, F. and Ghaderi, A. (2016) 'Development and evaluation of a Brief Motivational Interviewing training for exercise referral R.N.s and physiotherapists in Sweden', *Patient Education and Counseling*, 99(4), pp. 571-579.

3. Borrelli, B., Hecht, J.P., Papandonatos, G.D., Emmons, K.M., Tatewosian, L.R. and Abrams, D.B. (2005) 'Smoking-cessation counseling in the home: a comparison of results from two studies', *American Journal of Preventive Medicine*, 28(2), pp. 119-127.

4. Brobeck, E., Bergh, H., Odencrants, S. and Hildingh, C. (2011) 'Primary healthcare nurses' experiences with motivational interviewing in health promotion practice', *Journal of Clinical[1] Nursing*, 20(23-24), pp. 3322-3330.

5. Britt, E., Hudson, S.M. and Blampied, N.M. (2004) 'Motivational interviewing in health settings: a review', *Patient Education and Counseling*,[2] 53(2), pp. 147-155.

6. Catley, D., Goggin, K., Harris, K.J., Liston, R., Williams, K., Ekshteyn, M., Nazir, N., Ellerbeck, E.F. and Ahluwalia, J.S. (2012) 'A randomized trial of motivational interviewing: cessation induction among

smokers with low desire to quit', *American Journal of Preventive Medicine*,[3] 43(2), pp. 174-181.

7. Cox, M.E., Yancy, W.S. Jr., Coffman, C.J., Ostbye, T., Tulsky, J.A., Alexander, S.C., Dolor, R.J. and Pollak, K.I. (2011) 'Effects of counseling techniques on patients' weight-related attitudes and behaviors: results from the CHOICE randomized controlled trial', *Patient Education and Counseling*, 85(3), pp. 369-374.

8. Dinardo, M.M., Wetzel, G.T., Shirali, G., Breddy, J., Denhoff, E.R., Fish, F.A., Johnson, B.A., Law, I.H., Lindauer, B.M., Pilcher, T.A., Stephenson, E.A. and Etheridge, S.P. (2016) 'Motivational interviewing improves medication adherence in adolescents with inflammatory bowel disease', *Inflammatory Bowel Diseases*, 22(4), pp. 903-908.

9. Emmons, K.M., Puleo, E., Mertens, A., Geller, A.C., Heeren, T., Rudsari, A. and Gloriel, G. (2005) 'Long-term effects of a technical assistance and training intervention to improve sunscreen intervention in pools', *Health Education & Behavior*, 32(3), pp. 353-366.

10. Finfgeld-Connett, D. (2010) 'Motivational interviewing: A review of its effectiveness for health behavior change', *Worldviews on Evidence-Based Nursing*, 7(2), pp. 71-79.

11. Frederick, A., Nikkel, L.E., MacLaren, J.E., Fernandes, K.A., Carter, J.A., Hughes, S., Lee, R. and Carter, R. (2018) 'Motivational interviewing skills for nutrition and dietetics students: A qualitative study exploring

student experiences', *Journal of Human Nutrition and Dietetics*, 31(3), pp. 372-379.

12. Gillam, E., Betschel, S.D., Weber, B.A. and Gifford, W. (2017) 'Motivational interviewing for behaviour change in primary immunodeficiency nursing: A feasibility study', *Journal of Nursing Management*, 25(8), pp. 649-658.

13. Hardcastle, S.J., Taylor, A.H., Bailey, M.P., Harley, R.A. and Hagger, M.S. (2013) 'Effectiveness of a motivational interviewing intervention on weight loss, physical activity and cardiovascular[4] disease risk factors: a randomised controlled trial with a 12-month post-intervention follow-up', *International Journal of Behavioral Nutrition and Physical Activity*, 10(1),[5] p. 40.

14. Hettema, J., Steele, J. and Miller, W.R. (2005) 'Motivational Interviewing', *Annual Review of Clinical Psychology*, 1, pp. 91-111.

15. Hoek, S.M., Verhaak, P.F.M., van Dulmen, S. and Francke, A.L. (2020) 'Motivational interviewing as applied in nursing: A realist review of the mechanisms through which it works', *Patient Education and Counseling*, 103(11), pp. 2184-2194.

16. Jelsma, J.G.M., van der Schans, C.P., Krijnen, W.P. and van Leeuwen, E. (2016) 'Motivational Interviewing during Occupational Therapy: A Randomized Controlled Trial', *Scandinavian Journal of Occupational Therapy*, 23(3), pp. 213-222.

17. Knight, K.M., McGowan, L., Dickens, C. and Bundy, C. (2006) 'A systematic review of motivational

interviewing in physical health care settings', *British Journal of Health[6] Psychology*, 11(Pt 2), pp. 319-332.

18. Lundahl, B.W., Kunz, C., Brownell, C., Tollefson, D. and Burke, B.L. (2010) 'A meta-analysis of motivational interviewing: Twenty-five years of empirical studies',[7] *Research on Social Work Practice*,[8] 20(2), pp. 137-160.

19. Madson, M.B., Loignon, A.C. and Lane, C. (2009) 'Training in motivational interviewing: A systematic review', *Journal of Substance Abuse Treatment*,[9] 36(1), pp. 101-109.

20. Miller, W.R. and Rose, G.S. (2009) 'Toward a theory of motivational interviewing', *American Psychologist*, 64(6), pp. 527-537.

21. Miller, W.R. and Rollnick, S. (2013) *Motivational interviewing: Helping people change*. 3rd edn. New York: Guilford Press. (Note: This is a foundational book reference, often cited).

22. Mitchell, S.E., James, A.S., Morton, S.C., Tighiouart, H., Lafrance, J.P., Weiner, D.E., Stark, P.C., Chew, P. and Sarnak, M.J. (2014) 'Motivational interviewing to improve adherence to a complex health regimen in CKD patients', *Clinical Journal of the American Society of Nephrology*, 9(9), pp. 1556-1563.

23. O'Halloran, P.D., Blackstock, F., Shields, N., Holland, A., Iles, R., Kingsley, M., Bernhardt, J., Lannin, N., Lange, B. and Taylor, N.F. (2014) 'Motivational interviewing to increase physical activity in people with chronic health conditions: a systematic review

and meta-analysis', Clinical Rehabilitation, 28(12), pp. 1159-1171.

24. Pollak, K.I., Alexander, S.C., Coffman, C.J., Tulsky, J.A., Lyna, P., Dolor, R.J., James, I.E., Brouwer, R.J.N., Manusov, J.R. and Østbye, T. (2010) 'Physician communication techniques and weight loss in adults: Project CHAT', *American Journal of Preventive Medicine*, 39(4), pp. 321-328.

25. Rubak, S., Sandbaek, A., Lauritzen, T. and Christensen, B. (2005) 'Motivational interviewing: a systematic review and meta-analysis', *British Journal of General Practice*, 55(513), pp. 305-312.

26. Scales, R. and Miller, J.H. (2003) 'Motivational techniques for improving compliance with an exercise program: skills for primary care providers', *Disease Management & Health Outcomes*, 11(1), pp. 37-50.

27. Schoo, A.M.M., Lawn, S., Rudnik, E. and Litt, J.C. (2010) 'Australian primary health care nurses' contribution to lifestyle risk factor management: is there a gap between expectation and reality?', *Australian Journal of Primary Health*, 16(1), pp. 68-74.

28. Smith, L.A., Lake, A., Websdale, A., Osborn, D.P.I., Killaspy, H., Johnston, E., Landau, S., Michie, S., Pistrang, N., Craig, T.J.K. and King, M. (2014) 'Motivational interviewing for medication adherence in people with schizophrenia: a randomized controlled trial', *Psychological Medicine*, 44(10), pp. 2177-2187.

29. Tait, C., Dempsey, J. and Beeney, L.J. (2015) 'Motivational interviewing training for clinicians for medication adherence: a systematic review', *Patient Education and Counseling*, 98(11), pp. 1357-1364.

30. VanBuskirk, K.A. and Wetherell, J.L. (2014) 'Motivational interviewing in primary care: a systematic review of efficacy', *Journal of Behavioral Medicine*, 37(4), pp. 768-780.

31. Vasilaki, E.I., Hosier, S.G. and Cox, W.M. (2006) 'The efficacy of motivational interviewing as a brief intervention for excessive drinking: a meta-analytic[14] review', *Alcohol and Alcoholism*, 41(3), pp. 328-335.

www.ingramcontent.com/pod-product-compliance
Lightning Source LLC
Chambersburg PA
CBHW071716090426
42738CB00009B/1793